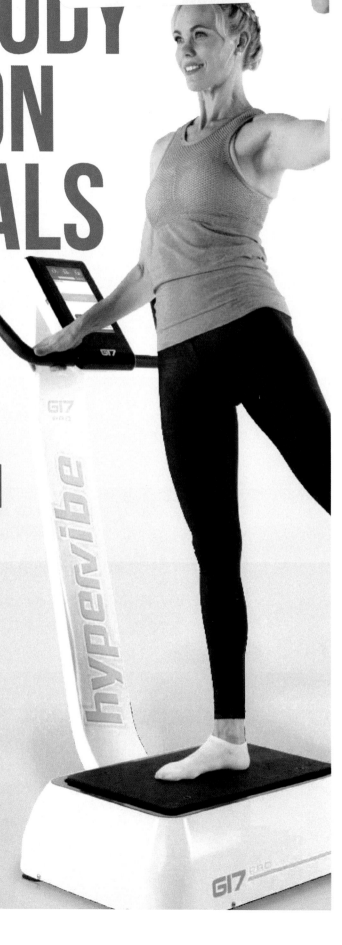

WHOLE BODY VIBRATION ESSENTIALS

PERSONAL EDUCATION COURSE & 60 DAY BODY TRANSFORMATION PROGRAM

INCLUDES ACCESS TO:

- 40 Exercise Programs
- Videos
- Meal Plans & Recipes
- Bonus Exercise Wall Chart

hypervibe

MW00952629

TABLE OF CONTENTS

60 DAY BODY TRANSFORMATION PROGRAM

EXERCISE GUIDES

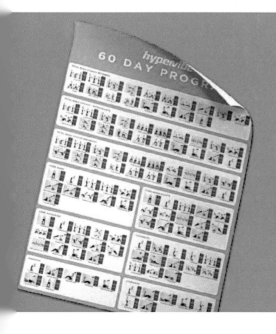

BONUS OFFER

GET THE FREE 60 DAY BODY TRANSFORMATION EXERCISE WALL CHART

◀ GET IT FOR FREE HERE

INTRODUCTION

Welcome to Whole Body Vibration Essentials, the personal education course designed for home users of Whole Body Vibration machines. If you are new to Whole Body Vibration or looking to expand your knowledge on this topic, this course has you covered.

In this course, we provide you with a basic understanding of the science behind Whole Body Vibration and how it can benefit your health. We then explain the different technologies and help you identify the type of machine you own so that you can follow exercise protocols correctly. Next, we will guide you through the basics of using your machine safely and effectively, including how to set your machine and the correct posture and positions to use during your workout. Finally, we will provide you with exercise programs and routines that you can use to get started on your Whole Body Vibration journey. These programs and routines are designed to help you achieve your specific health goals, whether you are looking to build strength, improve flexibility, or simply enhance your overall well-being.

By the end of this course, you will have a comprehensive understanding of Whole Body Vibration and how to use your machine safely and effectively. We hope that this knowledge will help you to achieve your health goals and lead a healthier, happier life.

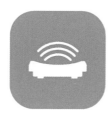

WHOLE BODY VIBRATION
VS VIBRATION THERAPY

Vibration as a therapy can be traced all the way back to ancient Greece when doctors would apply vibration to Greek Warriors for faster healing by sawing pieces of wood or plucking bow-like instruments. In more recent times, some of you may remember the old vibrating belt machines that were typically applied around the waist and violently shook your midsection. Although applying vibration to the body is the common theme among these examples and many others, it was not until the 1990's that modern day Whole Body Vibration was discovered and embraced.

The difference between Whole Body Vibration therapy and all other methods of vibration therapy that came before it, is the transfer of vibration to the entire body via the standing of a person on top of a vibrating platform. All other methods of vibration therapy transfer vibration locally to a body part and without being in a standing bodyweight loaded condition.

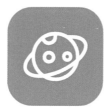

WHOLE BODY VIBRATION
AND THE SPACE PROGRAM

The concept of Whole Body Vibration has its roots in the Space Program, where scientists quickly learned that when astronauts were removed from the exposure to Earth's gravity, their bodies would quickly deteriorate. According to Dr Joan Vernikos, ex-director of life sciences at NASA, she walked into a nursing home one day and recognised that the conditions that she observed in the nursing home were not unlike the conditions being observed in astronauts returning from prolonged space flight e.g. poor balance, low bone density and muscle mass, decreased blood circulation etc. Apparently the theory that spaceflight caused rapid aging was not particularly popular with the astronauts!

This link between the returning astronauts and the elderly was not just a coincidence. In order to study the effects of zero gravity on astronauts, scientists from the space program have found that when subjects remain inactive in bed for extended periods of time here on Earth, they experience similar negative effects of being in a zero gravity environment. Anyone who has spent an extended period of time in a hospital bed would know the detrimental effect that this has on their health, with loss of muscle and bone etc. It seems that simply being on Earth does not mean gravity affects us equally.

In a standing position we experience the pull of Earth's gravity from head to toe, whereas when we are laying down, the pull of Earth's gravity is spread across our body and this results in less loading on our muscles and bones. These negative effects are not limited to being confined to a bed, spending excessive amounts of time sitting has been shown to have the same anti-gravity negative effects.

The observation that gravity has a relationship with our health gave birth to the idea that if a lack of exposure to gravity had a negative effect on the body, if somehow we could increase our exposure to gravity, would it have a positive effect on the body?

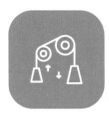

GRAVITY MACHINES

There are numerous examples of "gravity machines" we encounter throughout life, often they are associated with rides which involve fun and entertainment. Think of the rides at a carnival, a roller coaster, or the "gravitron". As the roller coaster drops down the steep decline, you suddenly feel very light, conversely as the roller coaster reaches the bottom of the decline and abruptly begins to incline, it feels as though your body has become much heavier. On the "Gravitron" your body is pulled towards the inner wall of the machine, making it very difficult for you to separate your body from the wall, its as if you were laying on the floor but your body weighs three times as much as it normally does, preventing you from getting up off the floor. These are examples of machines which use accelerating forces known as "g force", to increase (or sometimes decrease) your exposure to gravity.

By the same principle, when standing on a vibrating platform, as the platform accelerates your body in the upward direction (even though only momentarily), it also has the effect of increasing your exposure to gravity. When used in combination with a high g force setting, new users to Whole Body Vibration will often comment that they feel heavier.

Indeed, over 25 years of research has now demonstrated that while a lack of exposure to gravity has negative consequences for our health, increasing our exposure to gravity via a Whole Body Vibration machine has the opposite effect. Much of the early research on Whole Body Vibration came from the space program, where scientists would use Whole Body Vibration to improve muscle strength, bone density, and balance, just to name a few.

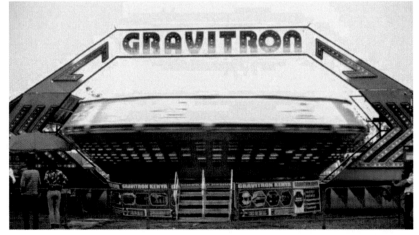

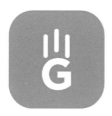

HOW MUCH GRAVITY?

Any Whole Body Vibration machine can produce vibration, and as we have briefly touched on, vibration applied locally can produce therapeutic effects, however, Whole Body Vibration machines often differ dramatically in their vibration settings and the resulting amount of g force they can produce. When g force levels on a Whole Body Vibration machine are set too low, they will not create enough stress to activate muscles, which is the key to building stronger muscles and bones.

Consider if you went to a carnival to ride the Gravitron, but it only operated at about half the speed at which it normally operates, below the speed necessary to stick you to the inner wall. Yes it looks like a Gravitron machine and it spins like one, but it's not really giving you the intended Gravitron experience. Likewise, when the g settings are too low on a Whole Body Vibration machine, you are not getting the outcomes that were intended via the Space program research.

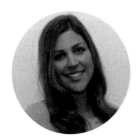

The vertical acceleration threshold that is required to significantly increase the sEMG activity of the lower limb muscles is around 1.8G.

DR. KARIN LIENHARD
UNIVERSITY OF CALGARY

Relationship Between Lower Limb Muscle Activity and Pltaform Acceleration During Whole Body Vibration, Lienhard et al. 2015

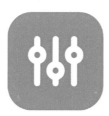

WHOLE BODY VIBRATION MACHINE SETTINGS

Read any of the +2000 scientific research studies involving Whole Body Vibration, and you will see the scientists create an exercise protocol for their experiment. This protocol is documented carefully, so that health professionals and other researchers can reproduce the protocol in order to repeat the experiment for themselves. Included in these protocols are vibration measurements of frequency, amplitude and g force, which are typically measured by the scientists with use of an instrument called an accelerometer.

Here is an example exercise protocol:

Total sessions:	**3 sessions per week for 12 weeks**
Exercise:	**8 x 1min squat per session**
Vibration frequency:	**25Hz**
Vibration amplitude:	**6mm**
Vibration G force:	**8g's**

All of these details are very important so that protocols can be reproduced by therapists and trainers wanting to achieve the same outcomes, or so that scientists can compare different protocols for better or worse outcomes. Likewise, for anyone using a machine at home, it also helps to understand these settings so that you can repeat the protocols that produce best outcomes.

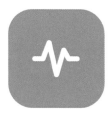

FREQUENCY

The frequency refers to how many times per second the platform vibrates or how fast it vibrates, measured in Hertz (Hz), and is controlled via the control panel on the machine. Frequency should be selected on the basis of your intended goal, e.g. for balance training use low frequency, for strength training use high frequency.

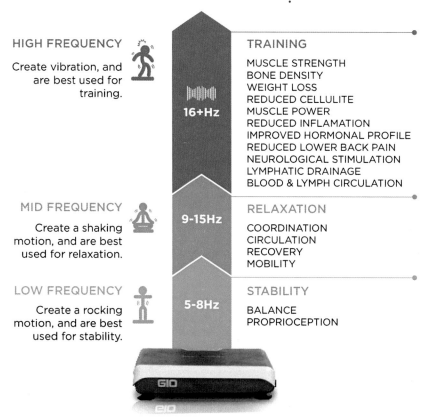

HIGH FREQUENCY
Create vibration, and are best used for training.

16+Hz

TRAINING
MUSCLE STRENGTH
BONE DENSITY
WEIGHT LOSS
REDUCED CELLULITE
MUSCLE POWER
REDUCED INFLAMATION
IMPROVED HORMONAL PROFILE
REDUCED LOWER BACK PAIN
NEUROLOGICAL STIMULATION
LYMPHATIC DRAINAGE
BLOOD & LYMPH CIRCULATION

MID FREQUENCY
Create a shaking motion, and are best used for relaxation.

9-15Hz

RELAXATION
COORDINATION
CIRCULATION
RECOVERY
MOBILITY

LOW FREQUENCY
Create a rocking motion, and are best used for stability.

5-8Hz

STABILITY
BALANCE
PROPRIOCEPTION

LOW FREQUENCY 5-8HZ

Low frequencies are usually only found in pivotal type machines (see Platform Motion) and when running at a low frequency, the term "vibration" is perhaps not an accurate description of the platform motion. At low frequency, the platform causes a slower rocking motion, and as a result there is a large degree of side to side, lateral motion in your body. Subsequently, much like standing on a rocking boat, most of your muscle contractions are made consciously to stabilize yourself.

 ## MID FREQUENCY 9-15HZ

Repetitive pulses of sufficient energy cause rhythmic muscle contractions. These muscle contractions create a strong pumping effect and result in a huge increase in peripheral blood flow, as well as lymphatic drainage. This can be particularly effective for those with poor circulation or swelling in the extremities. Mid frequencies are also usually only found in a pivotal type machines (see Platform Motion) and when running at a mid frequency, the term "vibration" is also perhaps not an accurate description of the platform motion. At mid frequency, the platform is still creating a large degree of lateral motion in your body, but with a noticeable higher intensity and rate of stimulation from the low frequencies, a shaking motion is induced. In fact, it is an industry known secret that mid frequencies, particularly in the 9-12Hz range, create a resonance in the machine and you will notice that the machine itself, tends to shake more in this range. The effects of shaking the body is well known in manual therapy techniques for the ability to induce muscle relaxation, improve blood flow to the limbs etc.

 ## HIGH FREQUENCY 16HZ+

Higher frequencies generate a faster platform movement and deliver more energy to your body, certainly higher frequencies can be described as vibration. At high frequency there is very little lateral motion, and although the intensity of the stimulation is increased, the feeling becomes less bumpy and smoother. With increased intensity, the higher frequencies cause the body to grow stronger and provide more stimulation. Due to the rapid rate of stimulation, most of the muscle contractions are involuntary reflexive muscle contractions.

IMPORTANT: Some machines display "speed levels" on their display, e.g. from 1 to 20, 1 to 50 etc. This should not be confused with frequency. Put simply, if you own a machine that starts at number 1 at the lowest setting, your machine is not displaying the frequency and you should ask the supplier what each number represents in terms of frequency, e.g. speed 1 = 3Hz. For more information, please see the following explainer

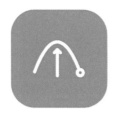

AMPLITUDE

The distance the platform travels up and down, measured in millimetres. On a lineal machine (See Platform Motion) amplitude is either fixed and can't be adjusted, or there will be a low amplitude and a high amplitude option on the control panel. On a pivotal machine (See Platform Motion) amplitude is controlled by simply moving your feet closer together or further apart. For reference points, Hypervibe has placed 3 amplitude positions on the platform, low, medium and high. Amplitude should be used to increase or decrease the g force intensity at any given frequency setting and should generally be used at a low position initially.

Larger amplitudes cause a greater amount of movement of muscles and joints and generate a stronger response from the organs controlling muscle reflexes. If however, the amplitude became so large that it caused you to bounce up and down off the platform, the exercise would become ineffective.

Small amplitudes are more comfortable for doing upper body work on the platform, however they will reduce the stimulation to your body and for lower body work could render the exercise ineffective. You should exercise with the largest amplitude you feel comfortable with.

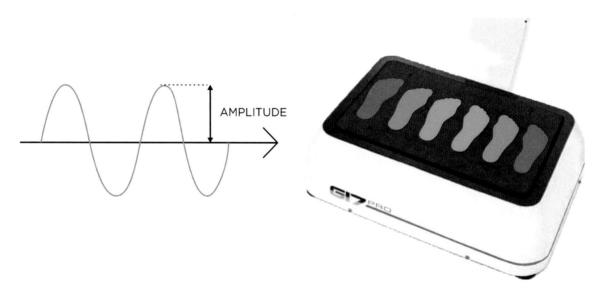

AMPLITUDE

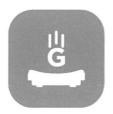

G FORCE

The gravitational force produced by the platform determines the intensity of the vibration, measured in g's, and is calculated by combining the frequency and amplitude settings, the higher both settings, the higher the g's, the lower both settings, the lower the g's. Hypervibe machines calculate the G force and show the value on the display, if you don't have a Hypervibe it is possible to calculate the G force of your Whole Body vibration machine settings using this calculator.

A lower frequency combined with a higher amplitude, can result in the same G force as a higher frequency combined with a lower amplitude.

For example:

A frequency of 40Hz with amplitude of 2mm = 10g
A frequency of 20Hz with amplitude of 4mm = 10g

This demonstrates why you can't judge the capability of a machine by just frequency or amplitude alone.

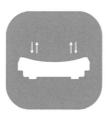

PLATFORM MOTION

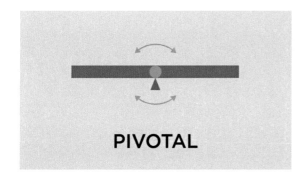

PIVOTAL

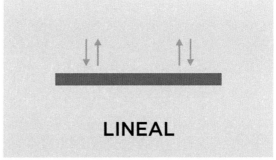

LINEAL

In addition to the above mentioned vibration settings, the platform of a Whole Body Vibration machine typically moves in one of two ways, either in a pivotal motion or in a lineal motion.

In pivotal vibration machines, the platform you stand on tilts around a central pivot point like a see-saw. The left and right sides alternate up and down while the centre remains fixed.

You can change the total distance your feet move up and down (other terms include 'displacement' and 'peak-to-peak amplitude') by moving them either closer or further away from the centre. The maximum possible distance varies from one machine to another but most are generally close to 10mm.

The pivotal platform movement mimics the natural rotation of the hips during walking and running which may activate a greater range of muscles and reduce vibration that occurs in the head.

A lineal vibration platform remains horizontal at all times with the entire platform moving up and down by the same amount.

Lineal vibration platforms typically have a small fixed peak-to-peak amplitude of 2mm or less. Some have 2 amplitude settings eg. low (1mm) or high (2mm).

Due to the platform moving the same small distance no matter where you make contact with it, upper body exercises on a lineal platform will be just as comfortable with a wide hand position as they will with a narrow one.

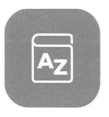

TERMINOLOGY

Unfortunately there are no universally agreed terms for these types of machines, so you will also find them labelled as follows...

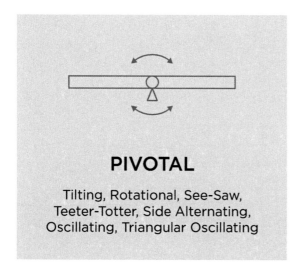

PIVOTAL

Tilting, Rotational, See-Saw, Teeter-Totter, Side Alternating, Oscillating, Triangular Oscillating

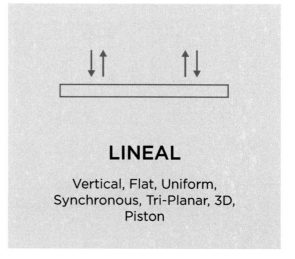

LINEAL

Vertical, Flat, Uniform, Synchronous, Tri-Planar, 3D, Piston

OTHER MOTIONS?

Over the years a few manufacturers have sought to create new platform motions in Whole Body Vibration machines, but nothing has been able to compete with the original methods described above. A couple of noteworthy examples would be:

1) A "stochastic" motion machine, where the user stands on 2 separate platforms and each platform vibrates randomly and independently of one another, in an attempt to replicate the forces experienced during downhill skiing. This method has shown some strengthening effects via research.

2) A "spiral/lateral" motion machine, where the platform vibrates horizontally instead of up/down. Sometimes also described as lateral pulsation, this method has failed to demonstrate any effect via research.

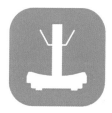

WHOLE BODY VIBRATION MACHINE TYPES

While there are a wide variety of brands and designs of Whole Body Vibration machines, they can be easily categorised into the following machine types.

 ## HOME USE - LOW FREQUENCY PIVOTAL

These machines are categorised according to their home use build, a pivotal platform motion, and also due to their lower vibration frequency capacity.

TYPICAL CHARACTERISTICS
- Price range: $100-$1,000
- Frequency range anywhere between 3-16Hz
- G force range from less than 1g up to approximately 6g
- Machine weight less than 40lb/18Kg (base only) or 80lb/36Kg (base + handles)

Due to their low frequency and subsequent low g force output, machines in this category are rarely used in scientific research and are supported for low to mid frequency range benefits only.

Note: It is common for machines in this category to be advertised with incorrect and exaggerated vibration specifications causing people to be misled about the performance.

Examples of machines in this category:

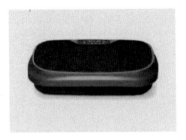

LIFEPRO WAVER

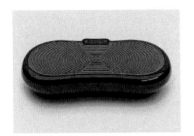

BLUEFIN

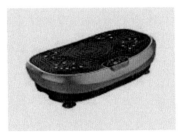

AVX

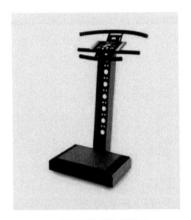

LIFETIMEVIBE

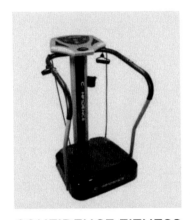

CONFIDENCE FITNESS

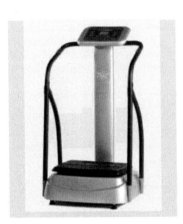

ZAAZ

 # HOME USE - FULL FREQUENCY PIVOTAL

These machines are categorised according to their home use build, a pivotal platform motion, and also due to their ability to produce a full range of vibration frequency.

TYPICAL CHARACTERISTICS

- Price range $1,000-$10,000
- Frequency range anywhere between 5-30Hz
- G force range from less than 1g up to approximately 15g
- Machine weight 60-80lb/27-36Kg (base only) or 90-130lb/41Kg-59Kg (base + handles)

With a full range of frequency and g force output, these machines are occasionally used in scientific research and are supported for low, mid and high frequency range benefits.

Examples of machines in this category:

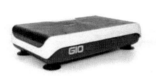

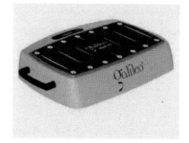

HYPERVIBE G10   **GALILEO S25**

 # COMMERCIAL USE - FULL FREQUENCY PIVOTAL

These machines are categorised according to their commercial build, a pivotal platform motion, and also due to their ability to produce a full range of vibration frequency.

TYPICAL CHARACTERISTICS

- Commonly used in scientific research
- Price range $4,000-$30,000
- Frequency range anywhere between 5-40Hz
- G force range from less than 1g up to approximately 30g
- Machine weight more than 90lb/41Kg (base only) or 140lb/64Kg (base + handles)

With a full range of frequency and g force output, and being of commercial grade, these machines are frequently used in scientific research and are supported for low, mid and high frequency range benefits.

Examples of machines in this category:

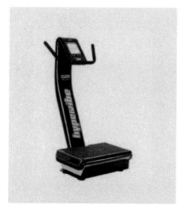

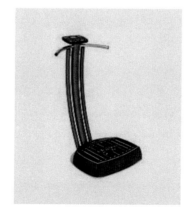

HYPERVIBE G25   **GALILEO FIT**

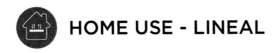 # HOME USE - LINEAL

These machines are categorised according to their home use build, lineal platform motion, and also due to their limited g force capacity.

TYPICAL CHARACTERISTICS

- Price range $100-$3,000
- Frequency range anywhere between 20-40Hz
- G force range from less than 1g up to approximately 4g
- Machine weight less than 40lb/18Kg (base only) or 150lb/68Kg (base + handles)
- No amplitude amplitude controls

Due to their low low g force output and limited control options, machines in this category are rarely used in scientific research. They are supported for high frequency benefits only, but with limitations due to low g force capacity.

Examples of machines in this category:

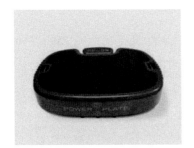 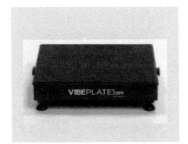 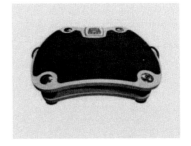

POWER PLATE PERSONAL   **VIBEPLATE MINI**   **BC VIBRANT HEALTH POWER 1000**

 # COMMERCIAL USE - LINEAL

These machines are categorised according to their commercial build, lineal platform motion, and also due to their higher g force capacity.

TYPICAL CHARACTERISTICS

- Price range $4000-$30,000
- Frequency range anywhere between 20-50Hz
- G force range from less than 1g up to approximately 15g
- Machine weight more than 140lb/64Kg (base only) or 240lb/108Kg (base + handles)
- Low or High amplitude option

With a large g force output, more control options, and being of commercial grade, these machines are frequently used in scientific research and are supported for high frequency range benefits.

Examples of machines in this category:

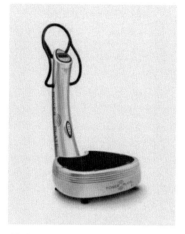

POWER PLATE PRO 5

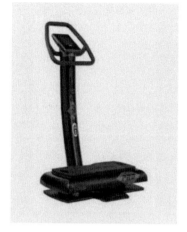

DKN XG10

 # OTHER CATEGORIES?

Generally speaking, attempts to create different technology have resulted in machines which do not work on the principles of Whole Body Vibration, i.e. to produce vibration mainly in the vertical direction to increase the supply of gravity to the body.

Some noteworthy mentions include:

Sonic/Sound technology machines, which use loudspeaker technology to drive a platform in a lineal motion. With use of sound technology, these machines allow a wide range of frequency control but the same technology is limited to small amplitudes, resulting in only low g force capability. There is no research supporting this technology.

Dual/Multi Mode machines, which typically allow a user to select from (low frequency) pivotal mode, or lateral mode, and sometimes both simultaneously. Although this might sound appealing, none of the modes available will produce the gravitational effects of high frequency pivotal or lineal machines. There is no research supporting this technology.

Low Intensity Vibration (LIV) machines, which use a lineal motion to produce micro amounts of vibration, usually at a frequency of approx 30Hz but with the amplitude of a fraction of a millimetre. Such a tiny amount of amplitude results in a g force of well under 1g. Such machines are marketed as being a safer option to increase bone density for the frail elderly, and there is some research supporting this effect via movement of fluid, however, due to their very low g force LIV machines do not provide the benefits of increasing the gravitational load.

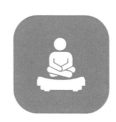

BENEFITS OF WHOLE BODY VIBRATION

STRONGER BONES

Bones become stronger when exposed to sufficient mechanical stress. Due to the muscle contractions and exposure to increased G-forces caused by a vibration machine, Whole Body Vibration has been shown to provide this kind of strength-inducing stress on bones.

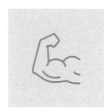

STRONGER MUSCLES

By increasing the pressure between your feet and the platform — which a Whole Body Vibration machine does by thrusting you upwards — the gravitational loading on your body grows, and forces your muscles to work harder. The stimulation a vibration machine places on your body is determined by the platform acceleration, or "G-force," where 'G' stands for 'Gravity'.

INCREASED CIRCULATION

Improving movement of blood and lymphatic fluid are things that vibration is particularly well suited to. It does so via the rapid up / down movement, with the corresponding increase / decrease of G-force causing the muscles to work. As the muscles increase their strength of contraction, it pumps blood through that area of the body — which means that circulation can be increased without straining the heart.

DECREASED BODY FAT

Hypervibe can stimulate your muscles at the same level of intense exercise, but without requiring significant effort on your part. By performing conventional exercises such as squats, lunges, push-ups, etc. on a Hypervibe machine, the increased forces on your body from the accelerating platform amplify the effect of the exercise.

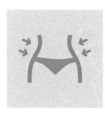

HORMONAL BOOST

Numerous studies have shown improvement in a variety of hormonal measures in adults. It is widely documented that strength training can facilitate hormonal improvements, and with Whole Body Vibration some of the research findings include:

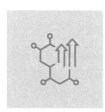

Cortisol levels : decreased by 32%

Testosterone levels : increased by 7%

Growth Hormone levels : increased by 360%

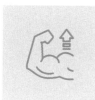

INCREASE MUSCLE POWER

Similar to the effects of plyometric training, but without the injury risk, Whole Body Vibration may be the most efficient and safe way to train the muscle system with this goal in mind. In research on muscle power, Whole Body Vibration — when administered in short, intense bursts — can quickly "kick in" the nervous system, resulting in an immediate and useful improvement in power (acute). In studies where it is administered differently, it has been shown to create longer-term (chronic) improvements in muscle power.

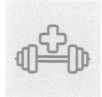

EXERCISE RECOVERY

Whole Body Vibration is an excellent tool to aid exercise recovery. Think of traditional recovery methods such as massage, stretching, and light exercise; Hypervibe can produce all of these effects simultaneously. Whole Body Vibration has been shown to enhance performance when used during recovery periods, and additionally, Whole Body Vibration is one of few methods that have been shown to be effective in reducing DOMS.

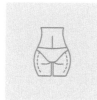

CELLULITE REDUCTION

The main problem with most cellulite treatments is that they focus on only one of the reasons for having it. For instance, draining your lymphatic system helps with fluid retention, but not fat burning. Deep tissue massage helps shift the fat cells, but not empty them. Exercise will empty them, but not shift them. Yet with the combination of these things provided by Whole Body Vibration, cellulite removal can be facilitated.

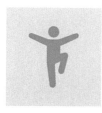

BETTER BALANCE

When you are standing on a vibration platform, the movement of the platform creates an unstable surface — but within a safe environment. This allows you to train your neuromuscular system to provide better stability and balance.

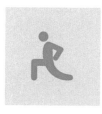

INCREASED FLEXIBILITY

The vibration or "oscillation" of the tissues caused by the rapid movement of the platform serves to both improve the mobility of the "fascia" that surrounds the muscles, as well as reduce the stiffness of the tissues that surround the joints. This allows the muscles and joints more freedom to move.

STRONGER PELVIC FLOOR

Whole Body Vibration has been shown to assist in strengthening the pelvic floor. Because of the functional movement pattern that the Hypervibe reproduces, simply standing on the platform while it vibrates forces the pelvis to move up and down in an alternating fashion (similar to walking). At lower intensities, this movement serves to release and relax tight tissue in the pelvic floor, while also stimulating the nervous system that supports the pelvic floor muscles. On the other hand, at higher intensities, the HyperVibe serves to improve the strength of the pelvic floor muscles, while also assisting with stabilizing the joints that connect the bones of the pelvic girdle.

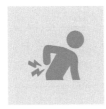

REDUCED BACK PAIN

Whole Body Vibration goes to the source of the pain by helping to strengthen your low back and core muscles, reduce muscle tightness, restore spinal motion, and improve postural alignment. All these things often contribute to the actual condition that caused the low back pain to occur in the first place.

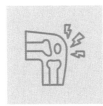

REDUCED JOINT PAIN

Joint pain is often treated with strength exercises because with sufficient muscle tissue surrounding a joint, the joint is better protected against irregular and aggravating movement. Research has shown that not only does Whole Body Vibration provide a pain free way to increase strength for people with arthritis, but it also reduces inflammation, as shown by a positive influence on inflammatory markers in the blood.

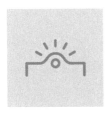

REDUCED SWELLING

Whole Body Vibration is one of the most reliable tools for assisting in the movement of blood and lymphatic fluid throughout the body. Similar to walking, but more efficient, the repeated forces placed on the body while the machine vibrates causes the muscles to contract at very rapid rates. The repeated contractions of the muscles enhance the natural "pump" mechanism of the lymphatic system, this helps it contend with any excess fluid.

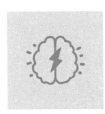

NEUROLOGICAL STIMULATION

Whole Body Vibration triggers a neural response by simply standing on the vibration platform and being exposed to the vibration. Studies have documented the reflexive neural response, which is triggered by the rapid stretching of the muscle when it undergoes the movement of the platform.

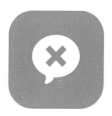

CONTRAINDICATIONS, PRECAUTIONS AND SIDE EFFECTS

From an occupational health and safety perspective vibration can be considered a negative that has deleterious effects on health. This occurs because of the low frequencies and long periods of repeated exposure in the workplace leading to exhaustion. However, for short periods on a whole body vibration platform there are no significant negative effects

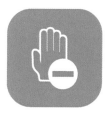

CONTRAINDICATIONS

Whole body vibration has been used around the world for over 30 years with no significant reporting of negative effects. However consideration of risk would be wise. Some conditions are discussed below

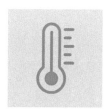

ACUTE INFLAMMATION/ INFECTIONS/ FEVER:
Whole body vibration causes peripheral vasodilation so may accentuate any acute inflammatory event or infection.

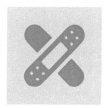

RECENT FRACTURES/ IMPLANTS/ SURGERY:
Recent Fractures/ Implants/ Surgery: Tissues take time to heal. Whole body vibration may overload hard and soft tissues during their healing phases. Once healing has occurred there are no restrictions.

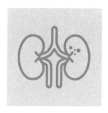

GALL AND KIDNEY STONES:
Gall and Kidney Stones: Whole body vibration may facilitate the passing of stones.

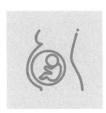

PREGNANCY:
There is no evidence of negative effects of whole body vibration on the mother or foetus but why take the risk?

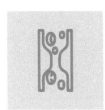

ACUTE THROMBOSIS:
Dislodgement of an embolus may lead to an infarct with catastrophic consequences.

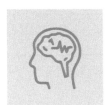

ACUTE EPILEPSY:
The vision of the rapidly vibrating plate may trigger an epileptic fit.

RECENTLY PLACE INTRAUTERINE DEVICES:
May be loosened by the vibration.

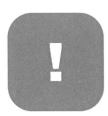

SIDE EFFECTS

Skin irritation: Skin lesions or blisters may occur on the skin in contact with the rapidly moving surface. Socks on feet, or a cloth on the platform will reduce any friction that may occur.

Diabetics may experience a quick drop in blood sugar levels dues to the high muscular activity so sugar lollies should be kept on hand.

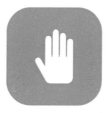

PRECAUTIONS

During the introductory stages when the experience is novel some side effects may occur. Nausea, dizziness, temporary drop in blood pressure and itching are usually harmless and are a sign of too high an intensity of exercise, especially in untrained users. Side effects usually disappear after the first few sessions.

For better preparation to the blood volume shift during whole body vibration the user may warm up fist. This is especially important for chronically hypoxic and/or geriatric users.

GETTING STARTED

PRACTICAL USE OF YOUR MACHINE

Before starting any of the exercise programs in this guide, it is important that you first understand some of the basics on how to use your machine, and become accustomed with its settings and operation.

DISCLAIMER

Hypervibe expressly disclaims liability for all damages and assumes no liability or responsibility for any loss, injury, or damage suffered by any person as a result of the use, misuse, reference to, reliance on or results obtained from any information, videos, audio or training manuals made available on this guide.

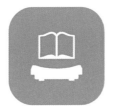

USING YOUR MACHINE WITH THIS GUIDE

When any vibration exercise program is designed, the following protocols should be included for each exercise:

- **Frequency** (adjusted on the control panel)
- **Amplitude** (adjusted by foot position on pivotal machines, or by control panel on lineal machines)
- **Time** (duration of the exercise)
- **Rest time** (rest duration after the exercise)

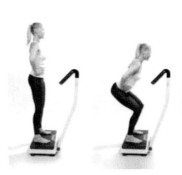
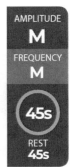

In our programs, time recommendations are shown (in seconds) inside the blue circle, and rest periods (in seconds) under the word REST. The rest time indicator should be considered a maximum recommended rest period, not a required rest period. If you don't need to use all of the rest time, please progress to the next exercise.

Because the frequency and amplitude settings of one vibration machine can differ significantly to another vibration machine, it is not possible to design specific vibration frequency and amplitude values that will be compatible with every vibration machine, so we refer to them as L, M, or H (Low, Medium, or High).

To understand what the recommended setting for L, M, or H is on your machine, you should follow the below steps:

Step 1 - Identify which type of machine you own (please refer to the guidance posted in the course section "Whole Body Vibration Machine Types"). If you are unsure, please find your brand and model and model of machine in the list here.

Step 2 - Use the recommended frequency and amplitude settings based on the instructions for your machine type listed below.

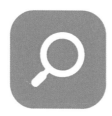

IDENTIFY YOUR MACHINE

 ## HOME USE - LOW FREQUENCY PIVOTAL

AMPLITUDE

Machines in this category may or may not have amplitude markers on the platform for your feet. Regardless, as we have already explained, amplitude is adjusted by moving your feet closer to or further away from the centre of the platform.

L	Stand with your feet close together in the middle of the platform.
M	Stand with your feet between the middle of the platform and the edge of the platform.
H	Stand with your feet out wide at the edge of the platform.

FREQUENCY

By design a low frequency pivotal is not able to produce high frequency vibration. However, when a high frequency is recommended in this guide, you are advised to set your machine to its maximum setting.

L	Set your machine anywhere between speed level 1 and 50% of the maximum speed level. For example, if your machine has 20 levels, set it between speed 1 and 10.
M	Set your machine anywhere between 50% of the maximum speed level and the maximum speed level.
H	Set your machine to maximum speed level

If a specific frequency is recommended in a video, you should consider whether the frequency mentioned is low, medium, or high according to the frequency chart and then apply the rules above. For example, if the video recommends using 20Hz, this is considered a high frequency and per the above rules, this means you should set your machine to maximum setting.

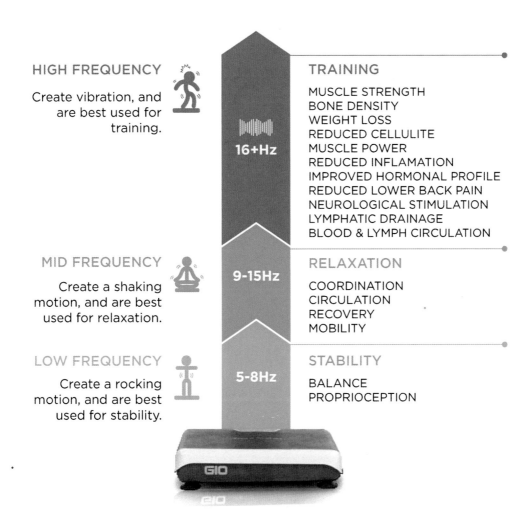

HIGH FREQUENCY

Create vibration, and are best used for training.

16+Hz

TRAINING

MUSCLE STRENGTH
BONE DENSITY
WEIGHT LOSS
REDUCED CELLULITE
MUSCLE POWER
REDUCED INFLAMATION
IMPROVED HORMONAL PROFILE
REDUCED LOWER BACK PAIN
NEUROLOGICAL STIMULATION
LYMPHATIC DRAINAGE
BLOOD & LYMPH CIRCULATION

MID FREQUENCY

Create a shaking motion, and are best used for relaxation.

9-15Hz

RELAXATION

COORDINATION
CIRCULATION
RECOVERY
MOBILITY

LOW FREQUENCY

Create a rocking motion, and are best used for stability.

5-8Hz

STABILITY

BALANCE
PROPRIOCEPTION

HOME OR COMMERCIAL USE - FULL FREQUENCY PIVOTAL

AMPLITUDE

Low: Stand with your feet at the low marker on the platform

Med: Stand with your feet at the med marker on the platform

High: Stand with your feet at the high marker on the platform

FREQUENCY

Low: Set your machine anywhere between 5-8Hz

Med: Set your machine anywhere between 9-15Hz

High: Set your machine to 16Hz or above

HOME OR COMMERCIAL USE - LINEAL

AMPLITUDE

Some lineal machines have a low/high amplitude control, while others do not. If you only have one fixed amplitude setting, you can disregard the following recommendations.

Low: Use the Low amplitude setting on your machine if available

Med: Use the High amplitude setting on your machine if available

High: Use the High amplitude setting on your machine if available

FREQUENCY

By design a lineal machine is not typically able to produce low or mid frequency vibration. However, when a low or mid frequency is recommended in this guide, you are advised to set your machine to its minimum setting.

Low: Set your machine at the lowest frequency setting

Med: Set your machine at the lowest frequency setting

High: Set your machine to maximum or no higher than 40Hz

If a specific frequency is recommended in a video, you should consider whether the frequency mentioned is low, medium, or high according to the frequency chart and then apply the rules above. For example, if the video recommends using 8Hz, this is considered a low frequency and per the above rules, this means you should set your machine to minimum setting.

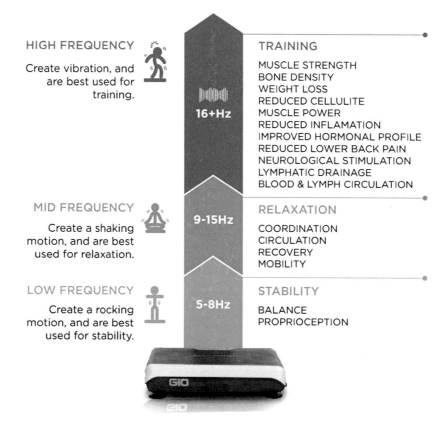

HIGH FREQUENCY

Create vibration, and are best used for training.

16+Hz

TRAINING

MUSCLE STRENGTH
BONE DENSITY
WEIGHT LOSS
REDUCED CELLULITE
MUSCLE POWER
REDUCED INFLAMATION
IMPROVED HORMONAL PROFILE
REDUCED LOWER BACK PAIN
NEUROLOGICAL STIMULATION
LYMPHATIC DRAINAGE
BLOOD & LYMPH CIRCULATION

MID FREQUENCY

Create a shaking motion, and are best used for relaxation.

9-15Hz

RELAXATION

COORDINATION
CIRCULATION
RECOVERY
MOBILITY

LOW FREQUENCY

Create a rocking motion, and are best used for stability.

5-8Hz

STABILITY

BALANCE
PROPRIOCEPTION

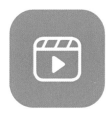

LEARNING THE BASICS: VIDEOS

! Remember, for best experience, it is best to wear a pair of socks only on your feet versus shoes.

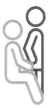

1) STAND OR SIT

Decide whether you have the ability to stand on the machine, or whether you would feel more comfortable from a seated position only. If you are only comfortable in a seated position, consider also some of the seated massage or stretching positions.

STAND

SIT

2) FOOT POSITION

If you are comfortable standing on the machine, learn about the importance of foot placement on the machine. It is important that you initially start with a low amplitude position, allowing you to feel the increase of frequency from the low position

only, and then if comfortable in low amplitude at high frequency, progress to a wider (medium) foot placement in the high frequency range.

NOTE: Amplitude is only adjusted by foot position on a pivotal type machine, users of lineal type machines should first experience low amplitude before switching to a high amplitude using their control panel.

3) FIRST EXERCISES

Try a 3-5 minute basic strengthening routine on the machine using high frequency and with low to medium foot placement. A few simple exercises such as standing, squats, rotations and spinal roll downs are some good exercises to try.

4) UPPER BODY EXERCISES

For people with a good level of strength, they may wish to try an exercise with their hands on the platform. Care should be taken with such exercises because the upper body does not have the larger muscles of the legs and glutes to absorb the vibration and additionally the vibration is transmitted more directly to the head.

Tips:

- Position your shoulders over your hands
- Pull your elbows in towards your torso

Initially try a kneeling push up and then place more body weight onto the platform to feel more intensity, progressing to a push up from your feet if desired. Unlike strengthening exercises from a standing position, it is recommended to try using a lower frequency initially.

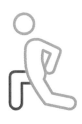

5) USING THE HYPERVIBE FOR STRETCHING

Stretching is a great way to start and/or finish an exercise routine or can be used alone to improve flexibility. There are a wide variety of stretching exercises and most people can find an exercise they are capable of doing.

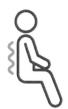

6) USING THE HYPERVIBE FOR MASSAGE

Massage is a great way to finish an exercise routine or can be used alone to improve blood flow, reduce pain etc.. There are a wide variety of massage positions and most areas of the body can be targeted.

60 DAY BODY TRANSFORMATION PROGRAM

GET THE FREE 60 DAY BODY TRANSFORMATION EXERCISE WALL CHART

◀ GET IT FOR FREE HERE

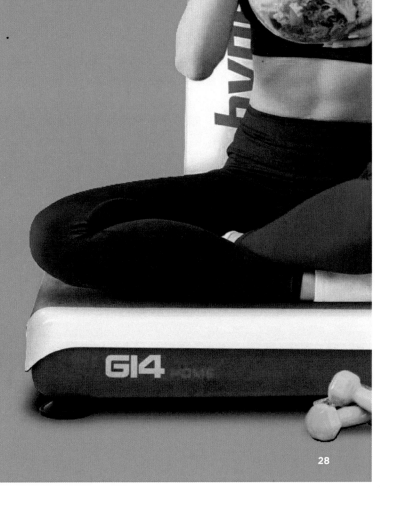

INTRO

Before beginning this program, we strongly recommend that you consult with your physician to assure the safety of the program for you. You should be in good physical condition and be able to participate in both aspects of the program (nutrition and exercise).

This program in no way represents a means to diagnose or treat medical conditions of any kind, or in determine the effect of nutrition or exercise on a medical condition.

You should understand that when participating in this or any other nutrition or exercise program, there is the possibility of injury or illness to occur. If you engage in this program, you agree that you do so at your own risk, are voluntarily participating in these activities, and assume all risk of injury to yourself. You also agree to release and discharge us from any and all claims or causes of action, known or unknown, arising out of our negligence.

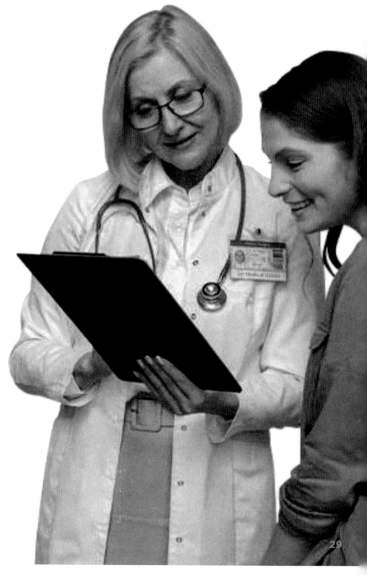

60-DAY PROGRAM

DAYS 1 - 7 | WEEK 1

DAY 1	DAY 2	DAY 3
Total Body Fitness Beginner	Flexibility	Total Body Fitness Beginner
Meal Plan 1	Meal Plan 2	Meal Plan 3

DAY 4	DAY 5	DAY 6
Lymphatic	Core Strength Beginner	Total Body Fitness Beginner
Meal Plan 4	Meal Plan 5	Meal Plan 6

DAY 7	notes
Massage	
Meal Plan 7	

DAYS 8 - 14 | WEEK 2

DAY 1	DAY 2	DAY 3
Total Body Fitness Beginner	Flexibility	Total Body Fitness Beginner
Meal Plan 8	Meal Plan 9	Meal Plan 10

DAY 4	DAY 5	DAY 6
Lymphatic	Core Strength Beginner	Total Body Fitness Beginner
Meal Plan 1	Meal Plan 2	Meal Plan 3

DAY 7	notes
Massage	
Meal Plan 4	

DAYS 15 - 21 | WEEK 3

DAY 1	DAY 2	DAY 3
Total Body Fitness Beginner Meal Plan 5	Flexibility Meal Plan 6	Total Body Fitness Intermediate Meal Plan 7

DAY 4	DAY 5	DAY 6
Lymphatic Meal Plan 8	Core Strength Intermediate Meal Plan 9	Total Body Fitness Intermediate Meal Plan 10

DAY 7	notes
Massage Meal Plan 1	

DAYS 22-28 | WEEK 4

DAY 1	DAY 2	DAY 3
Total Body Fitness Intermediate Meal Plan 2	Flexibility Meal Plan 3	Total Body Fitness Intermediate Meal Plan 4

DAY 4	DAY 5	DAY 6
Lymphatic Meal Plan 5	Core Strength Intermediate Meal Plan 6	Total Body Fitness Intermediate Meal Plan 7

DAY 7	notes
Massage Meal Plan 8	

DAYS 29 - 35 | WEEK 5

DAY 1	DAY 2	DAY 3
Total Body Fitness Intermediate	Flexibility	Total Body Fitness Intermediate
Meal Plan 9	Meal Plan 10	Meal Plan 1

DAY 4	DAY 5	DAY 6
Lymphatic	Core Strength Intermediate	Total Body Fitness Advanced
Meal Plan 2	Meal Plan 3	Meal Plan 4

DAY 7	notes
Massage	
Meal Plan 5	

DAYS 36 - 42 | WEEK 6

DAY 1	DAY 2	DAY 3
Total Body Fitness Advanced	Flexibility	Total Body Fitness Advanced
Meal Plan 6	Meal Plan 7	Meal Plan 8

DAY 4	DAY 5	DAY 6
Lymphatic	Core Strength Advanced	Total Body Fitness Advanced
Meal Plan 9	Meal Plan 10	Meal Plan 1

DAY 7	notes
Massage	
Meal Plan 2	

DAYS 43 - 49 | WEEK 7

DAY 1	DAY 2	DAY 3
Total Body Fitness Advanced Meal Plan	Flexibility Meal Plan 4	Total Body Fitness Advanced Meal Plan 5

DAY 4	DAY 5	DAY 6
Lymphatic Meal Plan 6	Core Strength Advanced Meal Plan 7	Total Body Fitness Advanced Meal Plan 8

DAY 7	notes
Massage Meal Plan 9	

DAYS 50 - 56 | WEEK 8

DAY 1	DAY 2	DAY 3
Total Body Fitness Advanced 2 Sets Meal Plan 10	Flexibility Meal Plan 1	Total Body Fitness Advanced 2 Sets Meal Plan 2

DAY 4	DAY 5	DAY 6
Lymphatic Meal Plan 3	Core Strength Advanced 2 Sets Meal Plan 4	Total Body Fitness Advanced 2 Sets Meal Plan 5

DAY 7	notes
Massage Meal Plan 6	

Week #1	Exercise	Level	Meal Plan #
❑ Day 1	Total Body Fitness	Beginner	1
❑ Day 2	Flexibility	n/a	2
❑ Day 3	Total Body Fitness	Beginner	3
❑ Day 4	Lymphatic	n/a	4
❑ Day 5	Core Strength	Beginner	5
❑ Day 6	Total Body Fitness	Beginner	6
❑ Day 7	Massage	n/a	7

Week #2	Exercise	Level	Meal Plan #
❑ Day 1	Total Body Fitness	Beginner	8
❑ Day 2	Flexibility	n/a	9
❑ Day 3	Total Body Fitness	Beginner	10
❑ Day 4	Lymphatic	n/a	1
❑ Day 5	Core Strength	Beginner	2
❑ Day 6	Total Body Fitness	Beginner	3
❑ Day 7	Massage	n/a	4

Week #3	Exercise	Level	Meal Plan #
❑ Day 1	Total Body Fitness	Beginner	5
❑ Day 2	Flexibility	n/a	6
❑ Day 3	Total Body Fitness	Intermediate	7
❑ Day 4	Lymphatic	n/a	8
❑ Day 5	Core Strength	Intermediate	9
❑ Day 6	Total Body Fitness	Intermediate	10
❑ Day 7	Massage		1

Week #4	Exercise	Level	Meal Plan #
❑ Day 1	Total Body Fitness	Intermediate	2
❑ Day 2	Flexibility	n/a	3
❑ Day 3	Total Body Fitness	Intermediate	4
❑ Day 4	Lymphatic	n/a	5
❑ Day 5	Core Strength	Intermediate	6
❑ Day 6	Total Body Fitness	Intermediate	7
❑ Day 7	Massage	n/a	8

notes

Week #5	Exercise	Level	Meal Plan #
☐ Day 1	Total Body Fitness	Intermediate	9
☐ Day 2	Flexibility		10
☐ Day 3	Total Body Fitness	Intermediate	1
☐ Day 4	Lymphatic		2
☐ Day 5	Core Strength	Intermediate	3
☐ Day 6	Total Body Fitness	Advanced	4
☐ Day 7	Massage		5

Week #6	Exercise	Level	Meal Plan #
☐ Day 1	Total Body Fitness	Advanced	6
☐ Day 2	Flexibility		7
☐ Day 3	Total Body Fitness	Advanced	8
☐ Day 4	Lymphatic		9
☐ Day 5	Core Strength	Advanced	10
☐ Day 6	Total Body Fitness	Advanced	1
☐ Day 7	Massage		2

Week #7	Exercise	Level	Meal Plan #
☐ Day 1	Total Body Fitness	Advanced	
☐ Day 2	Flexibility		4
☐ Day 3	Total Body Fitness	Advanced	5
☐ Day 4	Lymphatic		6
☐ Day 5	Core Strength	Advanced	7
☐ Day 6	Total Body Fitness	Advanced	8
☐ Day 7	Massage		9

Week #8	Exercise	Level	Meal Plan #
☐ Day 1	Total Body Fitness	Advanced (2 Sets)	10
☐ Day 2	Flexibility		1
☐ Day 3	Total Body Fitness	Advanced (2 Sets)	2
☐ Day 4	Lymphatic		3
☐ Day 5	Core Strength	Advanced (2 Sets)	4
☐ Day 6	Total Body Fitness	Advanced (2 Sets)	5
☐ Day 7	Massage		6

notes

ABOUT THE AUTHORS

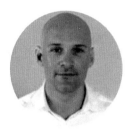

Gabriel Ettenson, MS, PT

Gabriel received his Master's Degree in Physical Therapy from Columbia University. He is both Colorado & New York State licensed and has been practicing for the past 15 years. Over his 15 years, he has completed numerous continuing education courses in manual therapy, musculoskeletal examination, soft tissue mobilization, ergonomics, and exercise prescription. Gabriel has also assisted in teaching for the doctoral program in Physical Therapy at Touro College in NY.

Gabriel's interest in WBV began 9 years ago when he came across an article on the subject. He then began using them personally, and eventually, with his patients in his Physical Therapy practice. Soon after he realized the tremendous benefits this technology offered, he went on to open Amplitude Vibration Studio in NYC with his business partner David Newman. Dedicated to Whole Body Vibration Training, Amplitude is one of the first Vibration Training Studios to be opened in the US.

Over the past 7 ½ years, Gabriel has used WBV technology with thousands of individuals of all ages and levels of health and fitness. He has presented the subject in the US and Canada to both professional fitness organizations as a variety of medical professionals. Additionally, he has had several articles published on the subject and has been featured on CBS news.

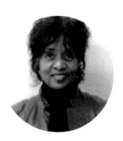

Cydya Smith, CHHC

Cydya graduated from the Institute for Integrative Nutrition where she studied more than one hundred dietary theories and a variety of practical lifestyle coaching methods. Her education allows her to help clients create a personalized "roadmap to health" that suits their unique body type and long-term nutrition and lifetime goals.

After being diagnosed with severe osteoporosis while she was in nutrition school, she was urged by her doctor to take medication and limit her activities. This was especially painful because she enjoyed an active lifestyle that included speed-walking, sky-diving, and learning to ride a horse.

After one year of living in fear of the side effects of the medication she was taking, she decided to take responsibility for her own health and researched ways to increase her bone density using alternative healing strategies. Her research focused on what could be done to mitigate her condition by using healing remedies found in real, non-genetically modified food & herbs, Whole Body Vibration, and meditation techniques for stress management. Her research paid off! Less than two years later she had increased her bone density (by 8.3% in one hip alone), lost weight, and improved her health overall. Additionally she has been featured on CBS news speaking about her results from WBV.

RULES OF THE 60-DAY BODY TRANSFORMATION PROGRAM

Nutrition Rules

To receive the optimum benefit of this exercise program, which includes losing weight, feeling healthier, and looking better, you must upgrade your nutrition plan and replace the "empty" calories from processed, denatured and genetically modified foods (containing GMO's) with nutrient dense **whole foods** and **healthy fats**. Do not focus on counting calories; focus rather on eating the right kind of calories, healthy fats, and nutrient rich foods at daily timed intervals.

Also, be sure to consult with your MD before beginning this nutrition program. This program is not meant to treat or diagnose any particular diseases and is to be done at your own risk.

Understand that any change to your diet is a learning process and learning to eat healthy means you must be proactive and do what is required to achieve your desired results. As Steven Covey says, from his best selling book, The Seven Habits of *Highly Effective* People, "Begin with the end in mind".

What do you wish to achieve? Remember... above all... You Are What You Eat!

Follow these primary rules for successful weight loss, weight management, and ultimate optimal health:

1. Plan your daily meals – Plan and prepare your meals at home.

If you fail to plan then you are planning to fail. Someone in the family has to invest time in planning and this person can also make use of the entire family to help – it's "One for all and all for one". Get everyone involved – then prepare and eat the majority of your meals at home. What you make for dinner you can take as your lunch the next day. This rule requires food shopping, menu planning and prepping. The Recipes section at the end of this guide will give you some great ideas.

2. Combine your food properly.

Protein with Veggies & Carbs with Veggies unless otherwise specified

3. Restrict sugars, fructose, GMO's & grains for this 60-day period.

This is a necessary strategy for better health in general, and especially so for those who intend to lose weight. Sugar addictions contribute to heart disease, diabetes, and obesity.

4. Increase consumption of healthy fats – especially Omega 3's.

Essential fatty acids are macronutrients that are not made by the body so they must be consumed through your diet. Most of us get enough of the omega-6's, but we all are lacking in the omega-3's, which slows down digestion by releasing a steady stream of glucose into your bloodstream. When your body does not get enough of these nutrients it needs, it sends out hunger signals and that cause cravings.

5. Consume lots of non-starchy vegetables, especially leafy greens!

These types of vegetables are wide in variety, low on the glycemic index, contain very little carbohydrates, and make a colorful presentation on your plate.

6. Add new foods, spices and herbs to expand your taste index.

Our palates deteriorate with age, so just as exercise keeps the body fit, exposing our palates to different and unusual foods, using new and exciting herbs and spices, can keep the sense of taste and flavor tuned.

7. Plan to exercise in the morning, and both eat and take your supplements within 30 minutes of exercising.

A plan to exercise in the am ensures the least likelihood that you will be prevented from doing it later in the day. The protein you need after exercise, you will get from your food so a meal after exercising is a must.

Calcium and magnesium, minerals that work synergistically in combination, will provide maximum benefit to bones, joints, and muscles if timely assimilated.

For example, magnesium is a crucially important mineral for a wide array of biological functions, including:

- Activating muscles and nerves

- Creating ATP - the energy molecules of the body

- Assisting the proper formation of bones and teeth

- Blood Vessel function

- Proper bowel function

- Helping digest proteins, carbohydrates, and fats

- Serving as a building blocks for RNA and DNA synthesis

- It's also a precursor for neurotransmitters like serotonin

Be sure that your MD approves of taking any supplements of course

8. Throughout the remainder of the day, eat every 3-4 hours.

Eating every three or four hours helps to release hormones that burn fat while also helping to regulate other hormones that make you put on weight. In addition, this helps to control cravings. Therefore, it is very important not to skip meals. Develop a routine that is right for you and stick to it.

9. If you don't like something, find a substitute!

There are vegan, gluten-fee, and vegetarian options you can explore in our "Substitutions" page.

10. Drink the right things. Avoid empty calories from beverages.

Pure filtered water mostly (at least 8 glasses a day and with a fresh squeeze of lemon juice if possible). Also, green tea, coconut water, almond milk, hemp milk, coconut milk, bone broths from grass fed and free range animals, and red wine (only 2 glasses per week please).

11. Keep a food diary on the blank pages of this booklet.

This makes and keeps you accountable. Be conscious of everything that you put in your mouth during this 60-day program. It all goes somewhere. Make it a game with the family and have everyone account from their food diary either daily or weekly. Use the calendar to count down the days and award nonfood prizes to yourself and family members

Additional Tips:

Quality over quantity has ever been the best value and the most enlightened choice. If your budget does not allow you to buy ALL of your food organic, the most important foods to buy organic are animal foods (meat, eggs, butter, cheese, etc.), especially if you and your family consume animal products regularly.

As far as other foods go, check out the Environmental Working Group's (EWG's) list of the "Dirty Dozen" fruits and vegetables that contain the highest amounts of pesticides and also their "Clean Fifteen" list of fruits and vegetables that are safe to purchase conventionally. You can download those lists from their website and carry them in your wallet.

Also, buy wild or locally caught seafood rather than farmed seafood for the same reasons.

By doing this, you'll discover that the nutrient density of the grass-fed and wild caught products will fully satisfy in smaller portions because of the richness of their flavor.

As you begin to expand your awareness about the quality of the food you eat, you may also discover yourself actively seeking opportunities to obtain quality. You can join buyers clubs and food coops to buy in bulk, or buy shares in local farmers clubs to offset the cost of both animal products as well as vegetables.

And... if these suggestions absolutely will not work for you, then read labels to choose food products carefully within your budget and follow the guidelines stated above. However, do try to limit your consumption of nonorganic animal products and GMO's during this 60-day period, and make some different protein choices, which are found on our "Substitutions" page. Finally, don't forget to diligently scrub and peel the skin from and wash all fresh fruits and vegetables, especially green leafy vegetables (use an organic vegetable wash).

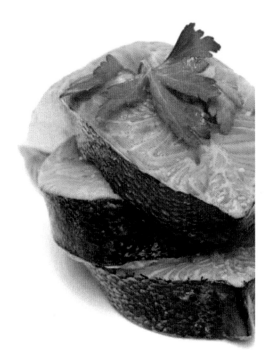

Exercise Rules

The following exercise rules are for general training on the Hypervibe as well as the specific programs within this guide. It is advised that you familiarize yourself with the rules below before training. Please consult with your MD before beginning any of these exercise programs. These programs are not meant to treat or diagnose any particular diseases and are to be done at your own risk.

1. Always minimize head vibration – Head vibration should be kept to a minimum. If any exercise causes excessive or uncomfortable amounts of head vibration, the following modifications can help:

- Add a small mat to the top of the platform. Be sure this mat is a non-slip mat.

- Slightly modify body position (i.e. bend knees a bit more when in standing positions).

- Reduce amplitude (move hands or feet to a lower number on the plate).

2. Never work beyond your capacity and stop IMMEDIATELY if you feel any pain.

3. The times given are meant to represent a goal. If you cannot complete an exercise at first, be patient and stop when you tire. Slowly you will succeed.

4. For exercises that include the need for balance, please use a chair or stool or the platform itself to provide additional stability if necessary.

5. If you have a history of vertigo or inner ear conditions, avoid positions with the head down towards floor.

6. Only follow the program calendar if you feel capable of the continuous progression. If you need to stay behind with a given exercise program, you will still benefit from the program. Take your time and do only what feels right.

7. Do not use shoes/sneakers unless absolutely necessary. Train with either bare feet or socks. If using socks, a rubber bottom is ideal. Otherwise, if you have regular socks, assure that your feet are stable when exercising.

8. Keep eyes open to avoid loss of balance.

9. Empty bladder before training for maximal comfort.

Potential Side Effects of Training:

10. Itching is normal. After first 3 sessions it will stop occurring.

11. "Floaters" indicate too much head vibration (repositioning needed)

12. Dizziness is typically a sign

a. Low blood sugar

b. Vestibular issues after a head down pose is held for too long.

13. Joint or tendon pain is a sign of overuse

14. Tingling may occur in feet after initial session. This will subside.

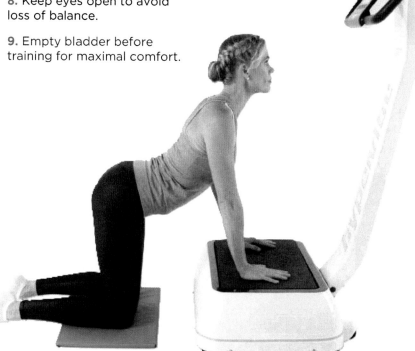

FOOD SUBSTITUTION

PROTEINS	SWEETENERS	GLUTEN-FREE	VEGAN
Tofu	Stevia (Packets or Liquid)	Quinoa	Beans, Lentils Legumes
Chia Seed	Coconut Nectar	Amaranth	Gluten-Free Breads
Hemp Seed	Coconut Palm Sugar	Beans, Lentils Legumes	Wheat-free Vegetable Protein
Greek Yogurt (Plain)	Birch Tree Sugar	Gluten free Breads	Miso
Whey Protein	Dates		Edamame
Almond Milk	Maple Syrup		
Hemp Milk	Raw Honey		
Nut Butters	Molasses		
Flax Seed	Artichoke Syrup		
Beans, Lentils, Legumes	Lucuma Powder		
Quinoa	Brown Rice Syrup		
Nuts	Barley Malt Syrup		
Miso	Xylitol		
Edamame			

*Do not use
Regular White Sugar
Nutra-Sweet
Splenda
Sacharrin
Aspertame
Or
other artificial
sweeteners

Highly Recommended Wild Protein Seafood Options:
Canned Sardines – Canned Dungeness Crab
Canned or Pouched Albacore Tuna or Salmon
Canned Mackerel
Canned Halibut

Feel free to substitute your lunch or dinner meal with the vegetable juice smoothie or with one of the other recipes in the Recipe section and be sure to use the recipe as a guide when you eat out.

EAT SMALLER PORTIONS FOR WEIGHT LOSS

Highly Recommended Wild/Grass Fed Protein Options:
Canned Sardines
Canned Mackerel
Halibut

HEALTHY OILS & FATS

Organic Extra Virgin, Cold Pressed Olive Oil

Coconut and Organic Extra Virgin, Cold Pressed Coconut Oil
(great for cooking because will not turn rancid at high temperatures)

Butter or Ghee made from raw, grass-fed organic milk

Raw nuts and seeds such as almonds, walnuts, pecans, brazil, sunflower, pumpkin

Organic, pasteurized egg yolks

Avocados

Wild Salmon
(high in Omega 3's)

Panseeda 5 blend raw oil

Raw nut or seed oils

Discontinue use of Vegetable and Canola oils - they are not on the NIH's (National Institute of Health's) healthy oils list and are most likely to contain GMO's.

SPICES & HERBS (Organic - Fresh & Dried)

Himalayan Crystal Salt* (fine or crystals)
Red Pepper Flakes
Turmeric
Cinnamon
Nutmeg

Ginger
(fresh, ground powder, crystallized)
Fennel
(Seeds and Ground)
Chili Powder
Cumin

Allspice
Cardamom
Black Pepper
Rosemary
Parsley
(flat leaf & curly)

Sage
Thyme
Dill
Cilantro
Tarragon
Mint

Celery Seed
Caraway Seed
Coriander
Sesame Seeds
(black and white)

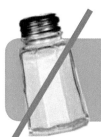

Discontinue use of regular, refined table salt because:

 Himalayan Crystal Salt contains 84 essential minerals that the body needs.

> The white color is due to bleaching and overall processing. The pinkish grayish tint is lost from the salt due to the removal of minerals and trace elements.

> Excessive intake of highly refined regular table salt is toxic for the body. The most common health problem caused by this salt is high blood pressure.

> Increased intake of salt reduces the ability of your kidneys to remove water, and the extra fluid puts strain on the blood vessels, thereby increasing blood pressure.

> Other problems that may result from high intake of refined salt are, arthritis, gout, red eyes, fluid retention, etc.

> Salt pulls water from the bloodstream, which disturbs normal water absorption process. This may lead to excessive thirst and constipation in a person.

ABOUT SUPER FOODS

Super foods are categories of foods that have powerful and unusual properties. Super foods are rich in nutrients, minerals and anti-oxidants that can protect your heart, slow down the aging process, improve your mood, enhance your brain function, improve your appearance, and help you perform at an optimum level.

Eating Super foods will help to limit low-grade inflammation in the body. Low-grade inflammation is the root cause of obesity, heart disease, osteoporosis, diabetes and many other ills that currently plague our society.

Super foods, such as dark leafy greens like Kale, Collards, Spinach, Chard, are high in anti-oxidants. Also high in antioxidants are beautifully colored Blueberries, Blackberries, Strawberries, and Goji Berries. Generally, the darker and more brightly colored a food is, the higher it is in antioxidants, meaning it is especially good for you.

Here is a list of my favorite Superfoods:

Olive Oil is a super food rich in phyto-chemicals found in fruits and vegetables that protect our cells against cancer and heart disease and it has a wonderful effect on your skin and hair.

Beans are good for your heart -- really! Beans are loaded with insoluble fiber, which helps lower cholesterol, as well as soluble fiber, which fills you up and helps rid your body of waste. They're also a good, low-fat source of protein, carbohydrates, magnesium, and potassium. Beans can substitute for meat or poultry as the centerpiece of a meal, but they also work as a side dish, or tossed into soups, stews, or egg dishes.

Dark Chocolate or Cacao is high in compounds that boost endorphins and serotonin, two of the best-known chemicals responsible for making us happy. It's also loaded with flavonoids, chemicals found naturally in plants that may help fight a wide array of conditions – including diabetes, strokes and heart disease – and flavonols, which can relax your blood vessels and thin your blood, lowering your blood-pressure numbers naturally. It may also help by curbing cravings for salt, sweet, or fatty diet-wreckers. To get the benefits of flavonoids, make sure to get dark chocolate that's at least 70% cacao.

Grapefruit contains a compound that can lower insulin, a fat-storage hormone, that can lead to weight loss. It's also a good source of protein, and because it's at least 90% water, it can fill you up so you eat less.

Green Tea hydrates like water, which can help fill you up and shed pounds. Plus, the antioxidants in green tea will up your fat burn and calorie burn. Spinach provides more than five times your daily dose of vitamin K, which helps blood clot and builds strong bones and also spinach reduces the decline in brain function associated with aging and protects the heart from cardiovascular disease.

Turkey - a 4-ounce portion of breast meat contains almost 50 percent of your daily selenium, a trace mineral that plays essential roles in immune function and antioxidant defense.

Kale contains all the essential amino acids and 9 nonessential ones and is unparalleled among dark leafy greens in nutritional density. Kale contains all 9 essential amino acids needed to form the proteins within the human body and compared to meat, the amino acids in kale are easier to extract. Kale is king of carotenoids. Its vitamin A activity is astounding. One cup contains over 10,000 IUs, or the equivalent of over 200% the daily value.

Apples contain quercetin, an antioxidant that may reduce your risk of lung cancer.

Shitake Mushrooms provides, in one-quarter pound serving, as much vitamin D as a glass of milk.

Berries especially Blueberries are among the best source of antioxidants and phytonutrients, are low in calories, and high in water and fiber to help control blood sugar and keep you full longer. Their flavors satisfy sweets cravings for a fraction of the calories in baked goods.

Salmon is a super food because of its omega-3 fatty acid content which helps protect heart health. Salmon is low in calories (200 for 3 ounces) has lots of protein, is a good source of iron, and is very low in saturated fat.

Eggs are nutritious, versatile, economical, and a great way for you to fill up on quality protein. Studies show if you eat eggs at breakfast, you may eat fewer calories during the day and lose weight without significantly affecting cholesterol levels. Eggs also contain 12 vitamins and minerals, including choline, which is good for brain development and memory.

Nuts are high in protein, heart-healthy fats, fiber, and antioxidants. They are healthful in small doses, and they can help lower cholesterol levels and promote weight loss. Nuts add texture and flavor to salads, side dishes, baked goods, cereals, and entrees.

Red wine, made with the dark skin and seeds of grapes, is rich in polyphenols, a type of antioxidant that includes resveratrol. Resveratrol, a natural plant compound, has antioxidant and inflammatory properties.

Sweet Potatoes are rich in beta-carotene and boasting 150% more antioxidants than blueberries, sweet potatoes are super high in heart-healthy vitamin and they're packed with vitamin C to keep your immune system strong.

Goat Cheese (fresh) and feta contain a fatty acid that helps you feel full and burn more fat. Look for cheeses labeled "grassfed," as those will have the highest content of this healthy fat.

Greek Yogurt has twice the protein of regular yogurt.

Flax Seed lowers blood cholesterol and reduces the risk of heart attack and also is a rich source of lignan, a powerful antioxidant that may be an ally against disease and certain cancers, especially breast cancer.

Steel Cut Oats are less processed than traditional oats and they're digested more slowly—keeping you full.

Chia seed has more calcium than a glass of milk, more Omega-3s than Salmon, and more antioxidants than blueberries. They also give you tons of energy but also won't keep you awake at night and are great for weight loss. Because they can absorb many times their size/weight in liquid, they are great for preventing dehydration during and after exercise. Add Chia seeds to your yogurt and in your post workout smoothies for the extra benefits you receive from them and because they fill you up.

Avocado contains healthy fats and nutrients such as oleic acid, lutein, folate, vitamin E, monounsaturated fats and glutathione among them. These can help protect your body from heart disease, cancer, degenerative eye and brain diseases. Avocados also taste great, are easily integrated into any meal – even a fruit smoothie. Add a half an avocado to smoothies to add creamy texture and a powerful nutritional boost, or enjoy an avocado half as a nutritious "side" to your morning omelet.

Sardines and other small cold-water fish, such as trout and mackerel, have less chance of being infused with mercury and pcb's. Best of all, they taste great, and are filled with what your body needs—Omega 3 Fatty acids. You must eat good fat to lose the bad fat your body is storing. You must consume foods high in Omega 3's, and in addition, you should also take a fish oil supplement. Omega 3's help you lose weight and they taste great.

Quinoa is a complete protein and is high in lysine (helps with the building of muscle protein and is useful for patients recovering from injuries and surgery). It is 35 on the glycemic index which makes it a good wheat or gluten replacement for those with allergies or blood sugar concerns.

Turmeric has been used for thousands of years for countless ailments. In recent years it has also caught
the attention of western researchers and there are many studies touting its many benefits. Some benefits include:

- Digestion and the liver (ulcers, diverticulitis, flatulence, leaky gut)
- Heart heath (high blood pressure, unhealthy cholesterol)
- Immune support (Cancer, colds and flu, bronchitis)
- Musculoskeletal strength and flexibility (joint disorders, arthritis, pain)
- Nervous system (pain, Alzheimer's Disease)
- Wound healing and healthy skin (eczema, psoriasis)
- Diabetes and menstruation difficulties

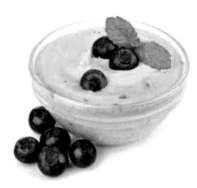

RECIPES

JUICES & SMOOTHIES

Green Vegetable Protein Juice Drink

Celery
Kale
Parsley
Cucumber
Spinach
Green Apple
Ginger
Sun Warrior Vegetable Protein
Coconut Water

Post Workout Smoothie

1½ Cups of cold Almond Milk
½ cup of cold Coconut Water
1 teaspoon Chia Seeds
Handful of baby spinach
1 slice of Fresh Ginger
½ small Avocado
Dash of Turmeric spice or
Turmeric Paste
1 scoop Organic Whey Protein from
grass-fed cows

Peach Berry Delight Smoothie

8 oz vanilla Almond Milk
2 tablespoons Blueberries
(Organic fresh or frozen)
5 Peach Slices (Organic Fresh or
Frozen)
1 slice of Fresh Ginger
Dash of Cardamom Spice and
Cinnamon
1 scoop Organic Whey Protein

Mango Magic Smoothie

8 oz Vanilla Hempseed Milk
4 oz Mango Coconut Water
1 tablespoon Lime Juice
2 tablespoons Raspberries (Organic
fresh
or frozen)
5 Mango Slices (Organic fresh or
frozen)
1 slice of Fresh ginger
Dash of Turmeric Spice
1 scoop Organic Whey Protein

Blackberry Ginger Smoothie

8 oz Hempseed Milk
4 oz Pomegranate Juice
4 tablespoons Blackberries (Organic fresh
or frozen)
2 slices of Fresh ginger
Dash of Cardamom Spice and
Cinnamon
1 scoop Whey Protein

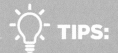 **TIPS:**

Buy vegetable juices from a health food store juice bar –(these are usually organic and will take the mystery out of doing this) unless you have your own juicer.

WHEN JUICING KALE, USE THE DARK LACINATO OR DINOSAUR KALE.

If using a blender, Vita-Mix, or Nutri-Bullet all vegetables and fruits will need to be chopped fine. Add filtered water and ice cubes to help liquify.

MAKE ICE CUBES FROM FILTERED WATER.

Slice Fresh Organic Ginger (peel and all) and store in plastic bag or container the freezer until you are ready to use it.

ADD STEVIA (SPARINGLY) TO YOUR TASTE IF NECESSARY.

Experiment with different spices to suit your own taste.

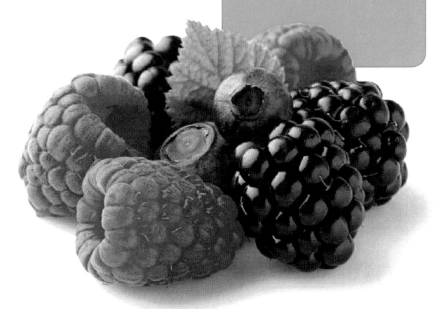

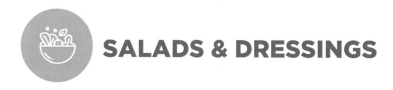

SALADS & DRESSINGS

Green Delight Salad

Mixed Greens
Mizuna
Romaine
Butter Lettuce
Cucumber
Mushrooms
Green Onions
Avocado (cut up)
Radishes
Canned Organic Tuna

Asian Chicken Salad

Mixed Greens
Mizuna
Romaine
Butter Lettuce
Cucumber
Mushrooms
Green Onions
Avocado (cut up)
Radishes
Canned Organic Tuna

Some recipes shared from the book
CLEAN by Dr. Alehandro Junger

Thai Cabbage Salad

3 cups finely shredded red cabbage
2 cups finely shredded green
cabbage
2 cups finely shredded napa
cabbage
2 cups bite sized cauliflower
1 avocado
½ cup minced fresh cilantro
¼ cup Living Harvest Organic Hemp
Oil
¼ cup extra virgin olive oil
¼ cup brown rice syrup
¼ cup nama shoyu or wheat free
tamari
3 Tbsp. umeboshi vinegar
1 inch fresh ginger, juice extracted
1 clove fresh garlic, minced
Generous pinch of chili powder.

Combine all ingredients in a large bowl
and toss gently. Set aside to marinate
for at least 30 minutes before serving

Apple Cider Vinegar
Salad Dressing

1/3 cup rice wine vinegar
1 teaspoon minced garlic
1 teaspoon minced ginger
2 tablespoons sesame oil
2 tablespoons agave nectar
1½ teaspoons chili powder
½ cup melted then cooled extra
virgin coconut oil
Shake ingredients and use
immediately

Asian Chicken Salad Dressing

1/3 cup organic agave nectar
1/3 cup organic extra-virgin olive oil
1/3 cup organic apple cider vinegar
1 clove garlic, minced
1 tablespoon spicy brown or Dijon
mustard

Combine vinegar, garlic and mustard
in a jar with lid
Mix well.
Add the olive oil, put the lid on the jar
Shake until the dressing is emulsified
Use what you need for your salad
Store the leftover amount for another
salad

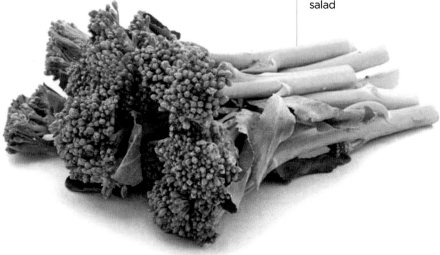

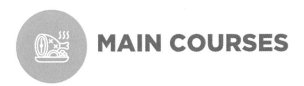

MAIN COURSES

Grilled Lamb Chops with Asparagus

4 lamb chops or 1 rack
Fresh rosemary (finely chopped)
2 cloves of garlic finely chopped
6 cloves of garlic (roasted)
1 tablespoon extra virgin olive oil
1 1tablespoon Dijon mustard
Ground salt (Himalayan Crystal Salt or Sea
Salt
Ground pepper
½ lb of baby asparagus

Trim asparagus.
Place asparagus in 1 inch of boiling, salted, filtered water and steam for 3 approximately 3 minutes until tender but not limp.
Drain and set aside
Make a paste of the olive oil, garlic, rosemary, and Dijon Mustard.
Brush lamb with the paste
Using high heat, grill, sauté, or broil lamb for 3 to 4 minutes on each side (for rare) longer if you prefer medium or well done.

Remove from heat and allow to lamb to rest.
Plate asparagus and arrange lamb chops.
Sprinkle with roasted garlic cloves.

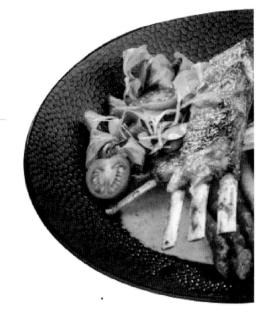

Moroccan Spiced Lamb Chops with Quinoa and Wilted Greens

4 lamb chops or 1 rack
Fresh rosemary (finely chopped)
2 cloves of garlic finely chopped
6 cloves of garlic (roasted)
1 tablespoon extra virgin olive oil
1 1tablespoon Dijon mustard
Ground salt (Himalayan Crystal Salt or Sea
Salt
Ground pepper
½ lb of baby asparagus

Prepare Quinoa with organic vegetable stock.
Mix all spices and salt in a small bowl.
Pat garlic all over the lamb chops, then sprinkle them with the spice mixture.
Heat oil in large skillet.
Add lamb chops, cook over moderate heat, turning once, 6 minutes for medium-rare -longer if you prefer.
Steam greens.
Transfer chops to two plates - garnish them with parsley and mint.
Serve with Quinoa and steamed greens on the side.

Grilled or Broiled Chicken Breast with Grilled Vegetables

2 (4 ounce) chicken breasts
3 tablespoons Olive oil
1 zucchini cut diagonally into 6 pieces
1 yellow squash cut diagonally into 6 pieces
1 portobello mushroom cut in half
1 teaspoon nama shoyu or wheat free tamari
6 asparagus spears trimmed and sliced
4 scallions

Combine nama shoyu or tamari and 1 tablespoon of the olive oil and marinate mushrooms in a bowl.
Place all vegetables except mushrooms in another small bowl - toss with 1 tablespoon olive oil, salt, and pepper.
Heat the grill or broiler to high.
Brush the chicken with 1 tablespoon of olive oil - season lightly with salt and pepper.
Grill or broil vegetables about 1½ minute on each side—set aside.
Grill Portobello mushrooms pieces for 2 minutes on both sides – set aside.

Grill Chicken breasts for about 3 minutes on each side.
Arrange all vegetables on plate.
Place chicken on top of vegetables.

Roast Chicken with Balsamic Vinegar, Garlic, and Rosemary Wild Rice Pilaf

2 (4 ounce) chicken breasts with skin
2 gloves garlic, sliced lengthwise
1½ cups of balsamic vinegar
2 tablespoons minced rosemary
22 tablespoons extra virgin olive oil
1 teaspoon salt (Himalayan Crystal or Sea Salt)
2 cups cooked wild rice made with vegetable stock
2 scallions thinly sliced
¼ cup chopped cilantro
¼ cup chopped fresh mint
½ cup of sunflower seeds, soaked for 2 hours

Cook chicken breasts with skin on for flavor them remove skin before eating Heat oven to 425 degrees.
In a small saucepan, reduce balsamic vinegar by simmering and stirring occasionally until it becomes the consistency of a syrup.
Add garlic and rosemary and simmer for 2 minutes more – set aside.
Brush chicken breasts with olive oil and salt.
Place on baking tray and roast in oven for 10 minutes.
Brush with generous amounts of balsamic mixture.
Turn the oven down to 375 degrees and roast for a further 10 minutes.

Brush again with balsamic mixture and cook 2 minutes more.
Remove from oven and let cool slightly, remove skins and thinly slice.
To make the pilaf, place the chicken, wild rice, scallions, cilantro, mint, and sunflower seeds in a bowl.Mix together and season with salt and pepper.

Depending on the season, you may want to serve this as room temperature or warm.
Soaking sunflower seeds activates the enzymes making the seeds easier to digest.

Stir-fry Vegetables and Chicken with Buckwheat Noodles

1 packet of buckwheat noodles (to make 2
cups when cooked)
1 teaspoon salt (Himalayan Crystal or Sea Salt)
l teaspoon sesame oil
2 carrots thinly sliced on the diagonal
1 cup of broccoli florets
1 cup snap peas
1 cup baby bok choy, sliced lengthwise
1 cup zucchini thinly sliced on the diagonal
1 scallion sliced into 2 inch pieces

Boil 6 cups of salted, filtered water in a large pot.
Add noodles, reduce heat slightly, and boil for about 3 minutes or until tender (but not limp).
Place noodles in colander and rinse thoroughly in cold water.
Drain water completely, toss lightly in the sesame oil – set aside.
Heat a heavy skillet and add olive oil. Keep on high heat .
Add garlic and ginger for 1 minute – stir with wooden spoon.
Add the rest of the vegetables (except snap peas) a little at a time to keep heat up.

Toss, flip or use wooden spoon to coat vegetables and prevent scorching.
Add nama shoyu and 2 tablespoons filtered water.
Finally add snap peas – stir - cook for 1 minute.
Garnish with fresh cilantro.
Serve sliced chicken breasts on the side.

Quinoa Salad with Chicken and Mixed Greens

2 cups cooked and cooled black quinoa
2 (4 ounce) chicken breasts, grilled or poached
and thinly sliced
1 tablespoon chopped parsley
¼ cup currants
¼ cup chopped raw almonds
½ cup dices carrots
¼ cup chopped mint

¼ cup chopped parsley
¼ cup lime juice
1 teaspoon agave nectar
½ teaspoon cumin
1 teaspoon salt
(Himalayan Crystal or Sea Salt)
½ cup olive oil

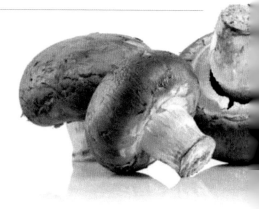

Roasted Wild Salmon or Cod with Cilantro Sauce, Black Quinoa and wilted Baby Spinach

MARINADE

1 teaspoon ground cumin
1 teaspoon salt (Himalayan Crystal or Sea Salt)
½ teaspoon ground ginger
½ teaspoon ground coriander
1/8 teaspoon ground red pepper
2 tablespoon Olive Oil (the best)

CILANTRO SAUCE

½ cup chopped fresh cilantro
½ cup chopped fresh Italian parsley
½ cup chopped fresh basil
2 large cloves garlic
Pinch of ground red pepper
¼ teaspoon salt (Himalayan Crystal or Sea Salt)
2 tablespoons fresh squeezed organic lemon juice
¼ cup extra virgin olive oil

Marinate 2 pieces of Salmon or 2 pieces of
Cod for 1 hour in marinade.
Combine all ingredients in a small bowl.
Brush both sides of fish.
Refrigerate until ready to cook.
Puree all cilantro sauce ingredients in blender and blend.
Preheat oven to 425 degrees.
Heat a large cast iron or oven-proof skillet over medium high heat.
Add fish and cook for 2 minutes, turn and cook 2 minutes more.
Place skillet in oven.
Cook fish 10 minutes more.
Prepare Black Quinoa in vegetable broth
Lay baby spinach on top (in same pot) with cooked quinoa and allow to wilt from the steam.

Quinoa Primavera Pasta

1 box (2 cups) Ancient Harvest Quinoa Pasta
Shells
½ lb Asparagus
½ lb Broccoli
1 Large Leek cut up
¼ lb Mushrooms, sliced
1, 8 oz can Black olives (pitted)
Red & Yellow pepper, finely chopped
1, 8 oz can of wild, sockeye salmon

Steam asparagus and broccoli al dente. cut into 1/2" pieces.
Sauté mushrooms, black olives, red and yellow pepper and red pepper flakes .
Cook pasta and add to sauté. Add steamed vegetables and salmon .
Toss all together with:

¼ cup of Light Olive Oil
½ teaspoon red pepper flakes
2 large cloves of garlic (chopped)

Finish with chopped fresh basil-salt and pepper to taste.

Steel Cut Slow Cooked Oatmeal Breakfast Cereal – Crockpot

1 cup steel cut oats
3 ½ cups water
1 cup almond milk or unsweetened coconut milk
½ teaspoon salt
1 ½ teaspoons cinnamon
½ teaspoon nutmeg
1 teaspoon vanilla
2 tablespoons butter

Combine the oats and other ingredients in the slow cooker.
Cook on low setting overnight for approximately 8 hours.
Add preferred toppings and enjoy!

Quinoa Breakfast Cereal

Prepare quinoa according to package directions.
Use filtered water, or almond milk, or coconut milk, or hempseed milk.
Add dried fruit or nuts as desired.
Sweeten (lightly) with agave nectar or brown rice syrup.

Black Beluga Lentil Salad

1 package Trader Joes black beluga fully
cooked lentils
½ teaspoon cumin
¼ teaspoon turmeric
1 tablespoon freshly grated ginger
1 clove crushed garlic
Juice from one (extremely juicy) lime
¼ cup pineapple (small dice)
¼ cup olive oil
½ teaspoon salt (Himalayan Crystal or
Sea Salt)
1 cup small diced zucchini
1 cup small diced cucumber
¾ cup small diced carrots
¼ cup cilantro leaves (pulled off
steams and chopped)
¼ cup scallions
2 cups salad greens

Remove Lentils from package -
place in a bowl – set aside.

To make dressing:

Place cumin, turmeric, ginger, garlic,
lime juice, olive oil, and salt in glass
jar or food processor and shake or
process.
Add pineapple to this mixture last
so dressing will be chunky.
To assemble salad, put all
vegetables (except greens) in to
bowl with the lentils.
Add dressing,- mix well and let sit
for 5 minutes to allow flavors to
blend.
Serve on top of greens.

Thai Vegetable Salad Wraps with Almond Sauce

1 tablespoon almond butter
1 teaspoon grated fresh ginger
½ large lemon juiced
1 teaspoon apple cider vinegar
1 clove garlic
1 teaspoon nama shoyu or wheat free
tamari
Pinch of cayenne
1/3 cup filtered water
Nori sheets cut into strips 1/8 inch thick
by
2 inches wide
4 large romaine lettuce leaves
½ shredded Napa cabbage
1 carrot shredded
2 scallions, thinly sliced
6 snow peas, thinly sliced
1 cucumber, peeled, seeded and thinly
sliced

To make almond sauce, blend
together almond butter, ginger,
lemon juice, water, apple cider
vinegar, garlic, and nama shoyu, or
tamari until creamy. If too thick, add
more water.
Wash lettuce leaves, dry thoroughly,
crisp in refrigerator in paper towels.
Combine remaining ingredients,
except nori, in a bowl.
When lettuce has dried and is a bit
crisp, put one quarter of mixture
into each lettuce leaf and roll up.
Garnish with cilantro leaf and strips
of nori.
Serve on a platter.

Adzuki Beans and Brown Rice

1 cup dry Adzuki beans, soaked.for 2
hours
or use organic, additive free canned
beans
1 red onion, diced
1 cup diced carrots
½ cup diced celery
1 cup diced butternut or kabucha squash
1 kombu leaf, rinsed well (Kombu is a sea
vegetable)
1 tablespoon extra virgin olive oil
1 cup brown rice soaked
1 ½ cups of cold filtered water

Heat olive oil in a medium-size pot.
Sauté the onions celery, and carrots.
Add adzuki beans, kombu, and 3
cups of filtered water.
Bring to boil, reduce heat, and
simmer for about 40 minutes or
until beans are tender.
Set aside to cool.
Place rice in a pot with 1½ cups of
filtered water.
Cover and simmer until all water is
absorbed – about 30 minutes
(check it periodically).
Place scoop of rice in the middle of
a bowl.
Ladle adzuki beans over it.
Garnish with fresh herbs (you
choose – let the taste buds of your
imagination run wild).
The Kombu seaweed adds minerals
and nutrients – You can also use
Wakame if you prefer.

Soups

Black Bean Soup

1 tablespoon extra virgin olive oil
2 green bell peppers, stems and seeds discarded, finely diced
1 large onion, finely diced
2 cloves garlic, minced on a microplane grater
1 jalapeño or serrano pepper, stems and seeds discarded, finely chopped
1 teaspoon ground cumin
½ teaspoon dried chili flakes
1 chipotle chili packed in adobo, finely chopped, plus 1 tablespoon adobo sauce from can (optional)
1 quart homemade or low-sodium canned chicken broth
2 (15-ounce) cans black beans, with liquid
2 bay leaves
Himalayan Crystal Salt

Heat vegetable oil in a large saucepan over medium-high heat until shimmering.
Add peppers and onions and cook, stirring frequently, until softened but not browned, about 3 minutes.
Add garlic, jalapeño, cumin, and dried chili flakes and cook, stirring constantly until fragrant, about 1 minute.
Add chipotle and adobo sauce (if using) and stir to combine.
Add chicken broth, beans and their liquid, and bay leaves.
Increase heat to high, and bring to a boil.
Reduce to a bare simmer, cover and cook for 15 minutes.

Discard the bay leaves.
Use a hand blender to roughly puree part of the beans until desired consistency is reached. Alternatively, transfer 2 cups of soup to a blender or food processor and process until smooth (start on low speed and increase to high to prevent blender blow-out).
Return to the soup and stir to combine.
Season to taste with salt.
Ladle soup into individual serving bowls and serve immediately with cilantro leaves, sour cream, diced avocado, and diced red onion (as desired).

Lentil Soup

1 teaspoon extra-virgin olive oil
½ small onion, finely chopped
1 carrot finely chopped
1 celery stalk, finely chopped
1 garlic clove, minced
Coarse salt and ground pepper
14.5 ounces low-sodium vegetable or chicken broth
3/4 cup cooked lentils (from a 15-ounce can), rinsed and drained
2 teaspoons red-wine vinegar

In a medium saucepan, heat oil over medium.
Add onion, celery, carrot, and garlic; season with salt and pepper and cook, stirring occasionally, until onion softens, 3 to 5 minutes.
Add broth; bring to a boil and cook 5 minutes.
Add lentils and cook until soup thickens slightly, 3 to 5 minutes.
Stir in vinegar and season with salt and pepper.

3 Bean Soup

2 onions, chopped
2 cloves garlic, minced
1 teaspoon grated fresh ginger
6 cups water
1 cup red lentils
1 (15 ounce) can garbanzo beans drained
1 (19 ounce) can cannellini beans
1 (14.5 ounce) can diced tomatoes
1/2 cup diced carrots
1/2 cup chopped celery
1 teaspoon garam masala
1 1/2 teaspoons ground cardamom
1/2 teaspoon ground cayenne pepper
1/2 teaspoon ground cumin
1 tablespoon extra virgin olive oil

In large pot saute; the onions, garlic, and ginger in a little olive oil for about 5 minutes.
Add the water, lentils, chick peas, white kidney beans, diced tomatoes, carrots, celery, garam masala, cardamom, cayenne pepper and cumin.
Bring to a boil for a few minutes then simmer for 1 to 1 1/2 hours or longer, until the lentils are soft.
Puree half the soup in a food processor or blender. Return the pureed soup to the pot, stir and enjoy!

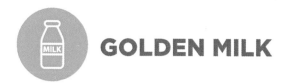

GOLDEN MILK

This recipe is in two parts. First make the turmeric paste.
To make the turmeric paste you'll need:

1/4 cup of turmeric powder
1/2 teaspoon of ground pepper
1/2 cup of water

Measure out the ingredients.
The additional pepper makes the turmeric more bio-available, meaning that you use less for better results.
At these measurements the pepper is about 3% of the mixture.
Next add the powders and the water to a small sauce pan and mix well.
Turn the heat to medium high and stir constantly until the mixture is a thick paste.

This won't take long!
Let this mixture cool and then keep it in a small jar in the fridge.

To make Golden Milk you'll need:

1 cup of milk (I use Hemp Milk)
1 teaspoon almond oil, ghee or coconut oil
1/4 teaspoon or more of turmeric paste
Honey or coconut nectar to taste

Combine all the ingredients (except honey or coconut nectar) in a saucepan and while stirring constantly heat the mixture until just before it boils.
Add honey or coconut nectar to taste.
Pour into cup and enjoy as a bedtime treat.

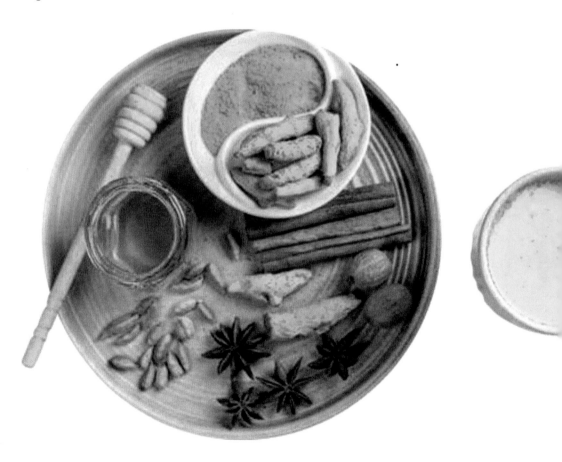

MEAL PLANS

MEAL #1

Pre Breakfast	Wake up – have 16 oz of lemon water to flush your body
Breakfast	½ Ruby Red Grapefruit 2 eggs scrambled with goat cheese and tomato 2 slices of Turkey Bacon Green Tea with Stevia
Mid Morning Snack-optional	16 oz of water – not optional ½ Apple (cut in slices) with almond butter
Post Workout Smoothie	Whey Protein Smoothie - 1 teaspoon Chia Seeds - *See Recipe*
Lunch	8 oz of water 3oz or 4oz Can of Tuna, Mackerel, Crabmeat, Sardines or Sockeye Salmon, packed in high quality olive oil Green Delight Salad – See Recipe 1/3 cup chick peas, sliced red, yellow, or orange cherry tomatoes Lemon Juice or Apple Cider Vinegar Dressing - *See Recipe*
Mid-Afternoon Snack	16 oz water 2 oz of organic sliced herbed turkey breast ½ Apple (cut in slices) with almond butter
Dinner	8 oz water Cup of Lentil Soup - *See Recipe* Chicken Breast - free range (broiled or grilled) sautéed spinach and shitake mushrooms with garlic Arugula salad, slice red onion, Red wine vinegar and olive oil
Evening Snack	1 piece of dark chocolate 4 almonds

MEAL #2

Pre Breakfast	Wake up – have 16 oz of lemon water to flush your body
Breakfast	2 slices of Turkey Bacon Cup of slow-cooked oats sprinkled with cinnamon, turmeric, 1 tsp flax seeds, and 2 tablespoons of frozen blueberries (they will thaw in the oatmeal) – dash of Stevia if you wish Cup Green tea
Mid Morning Snack-optional	16 oz of water – not optional 1 small pear 5 walnuts *If you don't have Mid- Morning Snack then have this for your Mid Afternoon Snack*
Post Workout Smoothie	Vegetable Juice Protein Smoothie – *See Recipe*
Lunch	8 oz of water 6 oz. broiled grass-fed beef or turkey burger (no bun) **or** 2 Large Romaine Lettuce Leaves to use as bun Large slice of organic beefsteak tomato Small mixed green salad with Avocado, white beans Olive oil and balsamic or apple cider vinegar
Mid-Afternoon Snack	16 oz water 2 oz of organic sliced herbed chicken breast 4 celery sticks with organic peanut or almond butter
Dinner	8 oz water Cup of mushroom soup 4 oz – broiled Salmon ½ cup steamed Kale Green salad with chopped tomatoes, cucumbers and red onion with olive oil, lemon juice and garlic
Evening Snack	1 piece of dark chocolate 4 almonds

MEAL #3

Pre Breakfast	Wake up – have 16 oz of lemon water to flush your body
Breakfast	½ cup of Blueberries 2 or 3 egg white omelet +1 yolk with organic pepper jack cheese and spinach Green Tea with Stevia
Mid Morning Snack-optional	16 oz of water - **not optional** ½ Apple (cut in slices) with almond butter
Post Workout Smoothie	Whey Protein Smoothie with 1 teaspoon Chia Seeds
Lunch	8 oz of water ½ Avocado Mashed with Lemon, Garlic Powder and Himalayan Crystal Salt on 1 slice of Whole Grain Toasted Bread Arugula Salad with chopped tomato, chopped red onion, 1/3 cup Black beans and splash of olive oil and lemon
Mid-Afternoon Snack	16 oz water 1 small pear 5 walnuts
Dinner	8 oz water Cup of Navy Bean Soup 6oz - grass fed flank steak (broiled or grilled) with sautéed/caramelized onions and dash of balsamic vinegar 1 cup steamed broccoli Chopped romaine lettuce salad, with sliced cherry tomatoes, chopped walnuts; dash Red wine vinegar and olive oil
Evening Snack	1 piece of dark chocolate 4 almonds

MEAL #4

Pre Breakfast	Wake up – have 16 oz of lemon water to flush your body
Breakfast	2 slices turkey bacon 1 cup of plain Greek yogurt sprinkled with cinnamon, turmeric, and chia seeds (add 1 drop Stevia) ½ cup of organic strawberries Green Tea
Mid Morning Snack-optional	16 oz of water - not optional ½ Apple (cut in slices) with almond butter
Post Workout Smoothie	Whey Protein Smoothie with 1 teaspoon Chia Seeds
Lunch	8 oz of water ½ cup of lentil soup - *See Recipe* 6oz can of crab meat with 1 tablespoon organic mayo mixed in with large green salad containing cucumbers, tomato, capers, and lemon
Mid-Afternoon Snack	16 oz water 1 hard-boiled egg ½ Apple (cut in slices) with almond butter
Dinner	8 oz water 6 oz broiled Halibut or Salmon Warm mixed bean salad with turkey bacon on wilted arugula, watercress or baby spinach Green tea
Evening Snack	1 piece of dark chocolate 4 almonds ½ cup of blueberries with lime squeeze and 1 drop vanilla stevia

MEAL #5

Pre Breakfast	Wake up – have 16 oz of lemon water to flush your body
Breakfast	Wild Mushroom and Goat Cheese Omelet 2 slices of turkey bacon Green Tea with Vanilla Stevia
Mid Morning Snack-optional	16 oz of water - **not optional** ½ Apple (cut in slices) with almond butter
Post Workout Smoothie	Whey Protein Smoothie with 1 teaspoon Chia Seeds
Lunch	8 oz of water Bowl of low sodium Vegetable soup ½ Turkey Bacon, Avocado, Tomato and Arugula sandwich on 1 piece of whole grain toasted bread 3 slices of pineapple
Mid-Afternoon Snack	16 oz water 2 oz of organic sliced herbed turkey breast 4 cherry tomatoes 2 brazil nuts
Dinner	8 oz water Cup of Lentil Soup – *See Recipe* 6 oz of roasted chicken breast ½ cup of roasted cauliflower with sweet green peas ½ cup chopped Zucchini, flat leaf parsley and tomato salad with olive oil and balsamic vinegar Green tea
Evening Snack	1 small pear 1 piece dark chocolate 4 almonds

MEAL #6

Pre Breakfast	Wake up – have 16 oz of lemon water to flush your body
Breakfast	½ Grapefruit 2 eggs scrambled with steamed kale 2 pieces Turkey Sausage Green Tea with Vanilla Stevia
Mid Morning Snack-optional	16 oz of water - **not optional** ½ Apple (cut in slices) with almond butter
Post Workout Smoothie	Vegetable Juice Protein Smoothie with 1 teaspoon Chia Seeds
Lunch	8 oz of water Asian Chicken Salad – *See Recipe*
Mid-Afternoon Snack	16 oz water 2 oz of smoked salmon 4 cherry tomatoes
Dinner	8 oz water ½ of Lentil Soup - See Recipe 6oz of grilled tuna steak with fresh tomato salsa with jalapeno pepper ½ cup of grilled zucchini, eggplant, red onion, orange or yellow bell peppers with light sprinkle of olive oil – dust with parmesan cheese Green tea
Evening Snack	1 piece of dark chocolate 4 walnuts

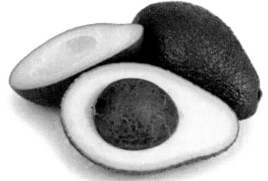

MEAL #7

Pre Breakfast	Wake up – have 16 oz of lemon water to flush your body
Breakfast	½ cup blueberries ½ cup of cottage cheese 2 slices Turkey Bacon Green Tea with Vanilla Stevia
Mid Morning Snack-optional	16 oz of water - not optional ½ Apple (cut in slices) with almond
Post Workout Smoothie	Vegetable Juice Protein Smoothie with 1 teaspoon Chia Seeds
Lunch	8 oz of water 3 or 4 oz Can of Tuna, Mackerel, Crabmeat, or Sardines packed in olive oil Green Delight Salad – *See Recipe* Lemon Juice Add chick peas, cherry tomatoes
Mid-Afternoon Snack	16 oz water 2 oz of organic sliced herbed turkey breast 4 celery sticks with almond butter
Dinner	8 oz water ½ cup of kidney bean soup Chicken Breast - free range (broiled or grilled) With grilled vegetables - *See Recipe* Romaine lettuce salad, sliced tomatoes, fresh basil leaves, olive oil, lemon juice and dusting of grated parmesan cheese
Evening Snack	1 piece of dark chocolate 4 almonds

MEAL #8

Pre Breakfast	Wake up – have 16 oz of lemon water to flush your body
Breakfast	½ Grapefruit Cup of slow cooked oats sprinkled with cinnamon, turmeric, chopped walnuts, 1 drop of vanilla Stevia 1 piece of Canadian Bacon or 2 pieces turkey bacon Green Tea
Mid Morning Snack-optional	16 oz of water - **not optional** ½ Apple (cut in slices) with almond butter
Post Workout Smoothie	Whey Protein Smoothie with 1 Teaspoon Chia Seeds
Lunch	8 oz of water ½ cup of vegetable broth Broiled Turkey Burger (no bun) 2 large Romaine lettuce leaves to use as buns or not 2 large tomato slices 1 slice of red onion
Mid-Afternoon Snack	16 oz water 5 oz of organic Greek yogurt with ½ cup blueberries and 1 teaspoon of Chia and Flax seed blend with cocoa and coconut
Dinner	8 oz water ½ cup of black bean soup - *See Recipe* 3 Avocado slices with 3 Tomato slices (dressed with garlic powder, lemon juice, high quality salt) Salmon Steak Grilled asparagus, or sautéed spinach or kale Green tea
Evening Snack	1 piece of dark chocolate 4 walnuts

MEAL #9

Pre Breakfast	Wake up – have 16 oz of lemon water to flush your body
Breakfast	½ Grapefruit 2 eggs scrambled with goat cheese, roasted tomatoes, and sprinkle of grated parmesan 1 piece of Turkey sausage Green Tea with Vanilla Stevia
Mid Morning Snack-optional	16 oz of water - **not optional** ½ Apple (cut in slices) with almond butter
Post Workout Smoothie	Whey Protein Smoothie with 1 tablespoon Chia Seeds
Lunch	8 oz of water Asian Chicken salad – *See Recipe* (If eating out- always order your dressing on the side)
Mid-Afternoon Snack	16 oz water 2 oz of organic sliced herbed turkey breast ½ Apple (cut in slices) with almond butter
Dinner	8 oz water 1 cup of lentil soup – *See Recipe* Quinoa pasta shells tossed with Roasted tomato sauce, black pitted olives, red pepper flakes and combination of chopped fresh flat-leaf parsley and basil. (add can of salmon, or tuna if you wish) Small Green salad with toasted pecans, blueberries– olive oil and balsamic Green tea
Evening Snack	1 piece of dark chocolate 4 almonds

MEAL #10

Pre Breakfast	Wake up – have 16 oz of lemon water to flush your body
Breakfast	2 slices turkey bacon 1 cup of plain Greek yogurt sprinkled with cinnamon, turmeric, and flax seeds (add 1 drop stevia) ½ cup of organic strawberries Green Tea
Mid Morning Snack-optional	16 oz of water - **not optional** ½ Apple (cut in slices) with almond butter
Post Workout Smoothie	Whey Protein Smoothie with 1 teaspoon Chia Seeds
Lunch	8 oz of water Thai Cabbage Salad – *See Recipe*
Mid-Afternoon Snack	16 oz water 1 hard-boiled egg 1oz or 1 slice herbed turkey breast ½ cup of blueberries
Dinner	8 oz water ½ Cup of Lentil Soup – *See Recipe* 5 oz Wild Salmon (broiled) over stir-fried vegetables (red peppers, onions, snow peas, broccoli, bok-choy, ginger, basil) teriyaki or soy sauce. Green tea
Evening Snack	1 piece of dark chocolate 4 walnuts

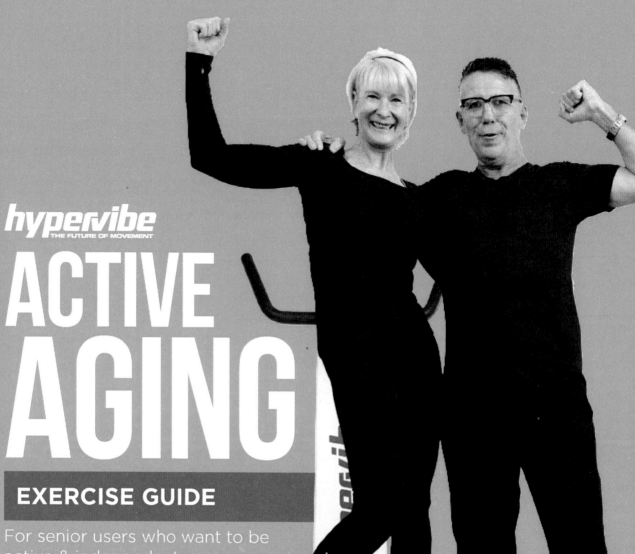

hypervibe
THE FUTURE OF MOVEMENT

ACTIVE
AGING

EXERCISE GUIDE

For senior users who want to be active & independent, move comfortably and be pain free.

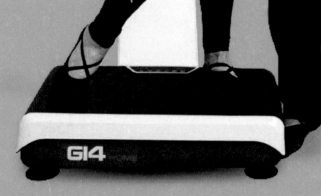

Introduction

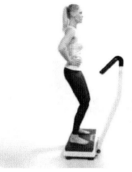
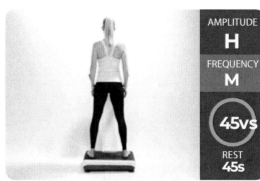

AMPLITUDE
M
FREQUENCY
M
45s
REST
45s

Normal Stance

AMPLITUDE
H
FREQUENCY
M
45vs
REST
45s

Wide Stance

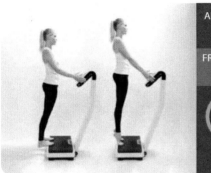
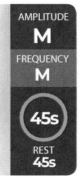
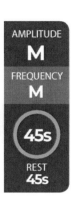

AMPLITUDE
M
FREQUENCY
M
45s
REST
45s

Calf Raise

AMPLITUDE
M
FREQUENCY
M
45s
REST
45s

Mini Squat

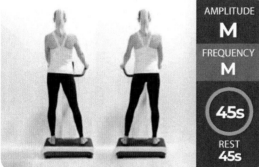
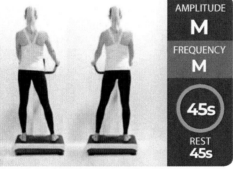
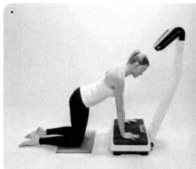
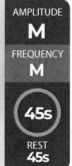

AMPLITUDE
M
FREQUENCY
M
45s
REST
45s

Standing Weight Shift

AMPLITUDE
M
FREQUENCY
M
45s
REST
45s

Shoulder Massage

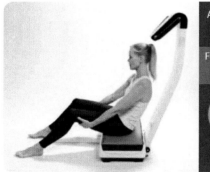
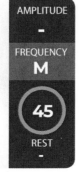

AMPLITUDE
-
FREQUENCY
M
45
REST
-

Seated Massage

Strong & Stable Beginner

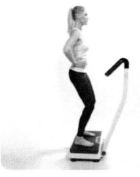
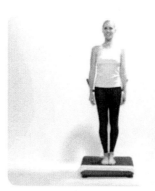
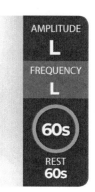

AMPLITUDE	H
FREQUENCY	L
60s	
REST	60s

Normal Stance

AMPLITUDE	L
FREQUENCY	L
60s	
REST	60s

Narrow Stance

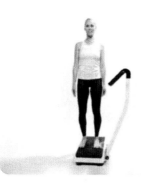
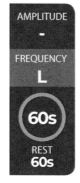
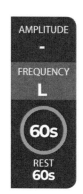

AMPLITUDE	-
FREQUENCY	L
60s	
REST	60s

Wide Side Stance

AMPLITUDE	-
FREQUENCY	L
60s	
REST	60s

Narrow Side Stance

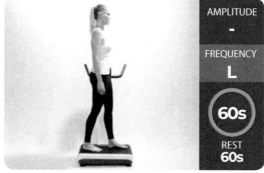
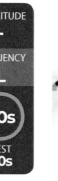
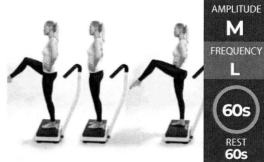

AMPLITUDE	-
FREQUENCY	L
60s	
REST	60s

Tandem Side Stance

AMPLITUDE	M
FREQUENCY	L
60s	
REST	60s

Alternating Knee Lift

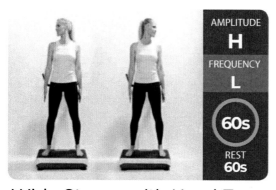
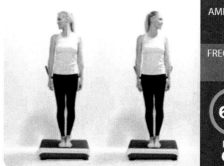
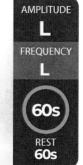

AMPLITUDE	H
FREQUENCY	L
60s	
REST	60s

Wide Stance with Head Turn

AMPLITUDE	L
FREQUENCY	L
60s	
REST	60s

Narrow Stance with Head Turn

Strong & Stable Beginner

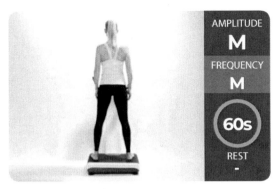

Lumbar Massage

Strong & Stable Intermediate

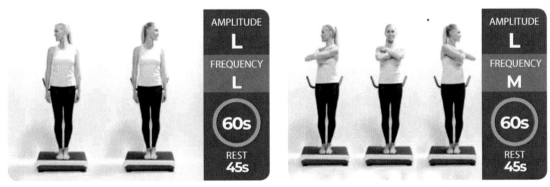

Narrow Stance with Head Turn   Narrow Stance with Rotation

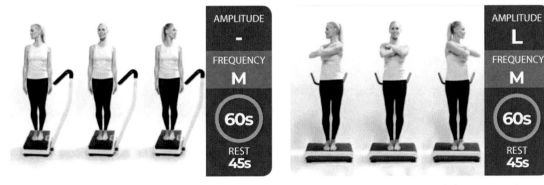

Narrow Side Stance with Head Turn   Narrow Stance with Rotation

Strong & Stable Intermediate

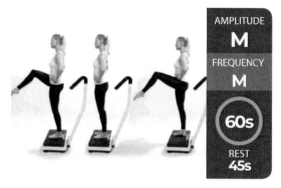

AMPLITUDE **M**
FREQUENCY **M**
60s
REST 45s

Alternating Knee Lift

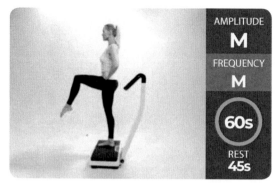

AMPLITUDE **M**
FREQUENCY **M**
60s
REST 45s

Single Leg Standing LEFT

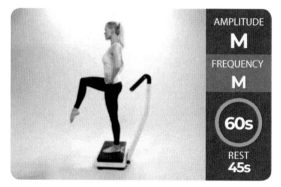

AMPLITUDE **M**
FREQUENCY **M**
60s
REST 45s

Single Leg Standing RIGHT

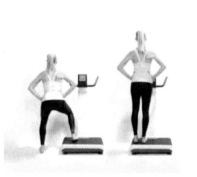

AMPLITUDE **M**
FREQUENCY **M**
60s
REST 45s

Step Up LEFT

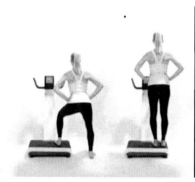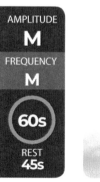

AMPLITUDE **M**
FREQUENCY **M**
60s
REST 45s

Step Up RIGHT

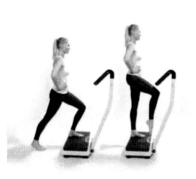

AMPLITUDE **M**
FREQUENCY **M**
60s
REST 45s

Step Up with Knee Lift LEFT

AMPLITUDE **M**
FREQUENCY **M**
60s
REST 45s

Step Up with Knee Lift RIGHT

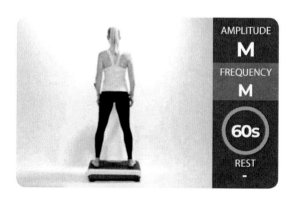

AMPLITUDE **M**
FREQUENCY **M**
60s
REST -

Lumbar Massage

Strong & Stable Advanced

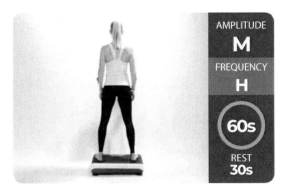

AMPLITUDE M
FREQUENCY H
60s
REST 30s

Wide Stance

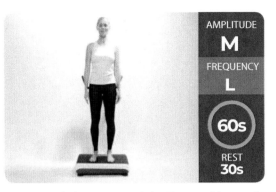

AMPLITUDE M
FREQUENCY L
60s
REST 30s

Normal Stance with Eyes Closed

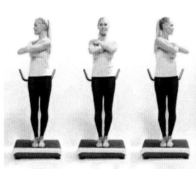

AMPLITUDE L
FREQUENCY H
60s
REST 30s

Narrow Stance with Rotation

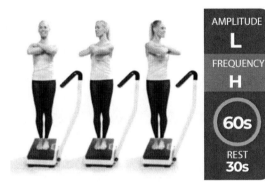

AMPLITUDE L
FREQUENCY H
60s
REST 30s

Narrow Side Stance with Rotation

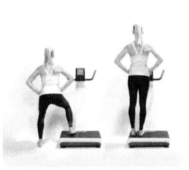

AMPLITUDE L
FREQUENCY H
60s
REST 30s

Step Up LEFT

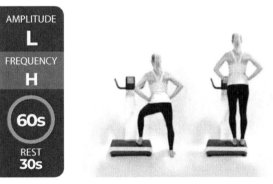

AMPLITUDE L
FREQUENCY H
60s
REST 30s

Step Up RIGHT

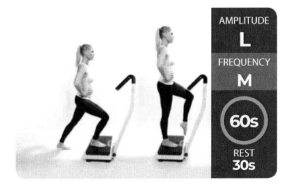

AMPLITUDE L
FREQUENCY M
60s
REST 30s

Step Up with Knee Lift LEFT

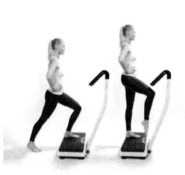

AMPLITUDE L
FREQUENCY M
60s
REST 30s

Step Up with Knee Lift RIGHT

Strong & Stable Advanced

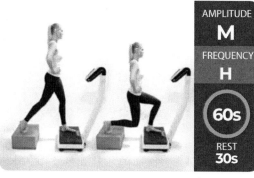

Lunge LEFT

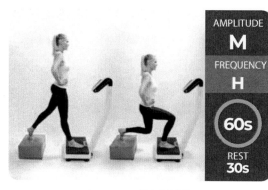

Lunge RIGHT

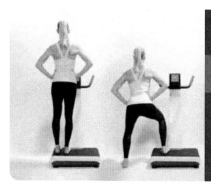

Lateral Step Up LEFT

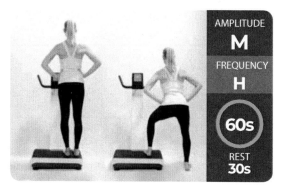

Lateral Step Up RIGHT

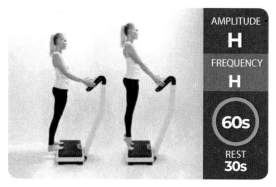

Calf Raise

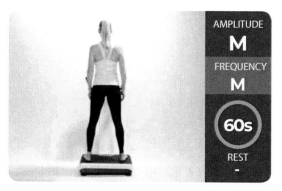

Lumbar Massage

Active Fitness Beginner

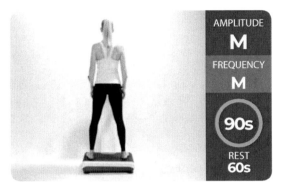

AMPLITUDE **M**
FREQUENCY **M**
90s
REST **60s**

Wide Stance

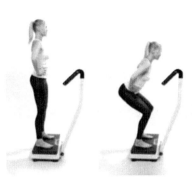
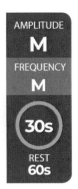

AMPLITUDE **M**
FREQUENCY **M**
30s
REST **60s**

Mini Squat

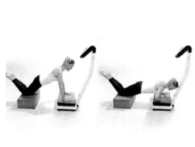

AMPLITUDE **M**
FREQUENCY **M**
30s
REST **60s**

Single Leg Knee Lift LEFT

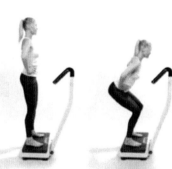
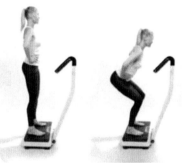

AMPLITUDE **M**
FREQUENCY **M**
30s
REST **60s**

Single Leg Knee Lift RIGHT

AMPLITUDE **H**
FREQUENCY **M**
30s
REST **60s**

Modified Push Up

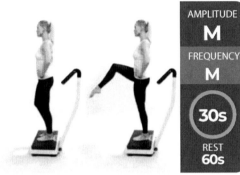

AMPLITUDE **M**
FREQUENCY **H**
30s
REST **60s**

Mini Squat

AMPLITUDE **M**
FREQUENCY **H**
30s
REST **60s**

Calf Raise

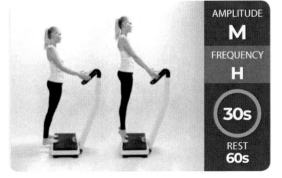
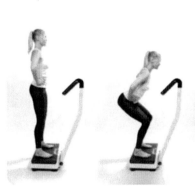
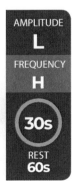

AMPLITUDE **L**
FREQUENCY **H**
30s
REST **60s**

Mini Squat

Active Fitness Beginner

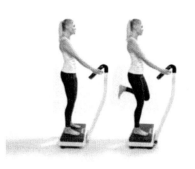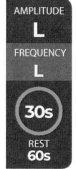

Standing Hamstring Curls LEFT

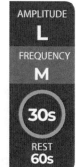

Standing Hamstring Curls RIGHT

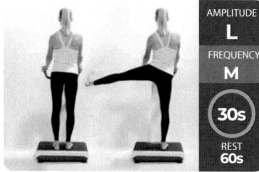

Hip Abduction LEFT

Hip Abduction RIGHT

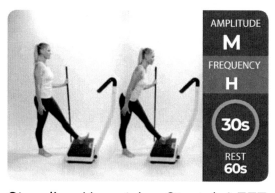

Standing Hamstring Stretch LEFT

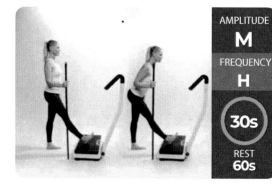

Standing Hamstring Stretch RIGHT

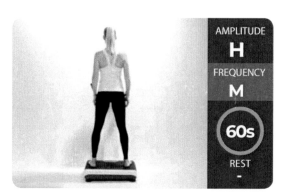

Lumbar Massage

Active Fitness Intermediate

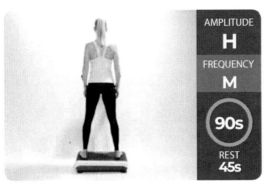

AMPLITUDE **H**
FREQUENCY **M**
90s
REST **45s**

Wide Stance

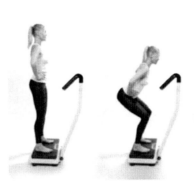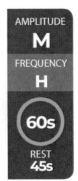

AMPLITUDE **M**
FREQUENCY **H**
60s
REST **45s**

Mini Squat

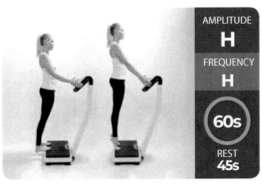

AMPLITUDE **M**
FREQUENCY **H**
60s
REST **45s**

Deep Squat

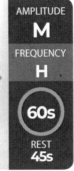

AMPLITUDE **H**
FREQUENCY **M**
60s
REST **45s**

Modified Push Up

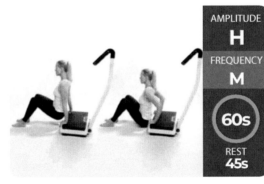

AMPLITUDE **H**
FREQUENCY **H**
60s
REST **45s**

Calf Raise

AMPLITUDE **H**
FREQUENCY **M**
60s
REST **45s**

Triceps Dip

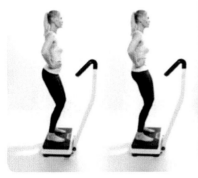

AMPLITUDE **M**
FREQUENCY **M**
60s
REST **45s**

Pelvic Tilts

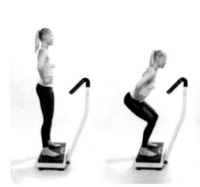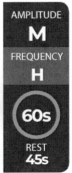

AMPLITUDE **M**
FREQUENCY **H**
60s
REST **45s**

Mini Squat

Active Fitness Intermediate

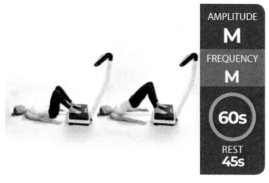

Bridge

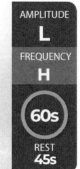

Hip Abduction LEFT

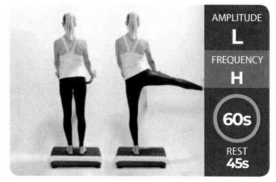

Hip Abduction RIGHT

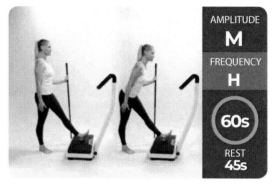

Standing Hamstring Stretch LEFT

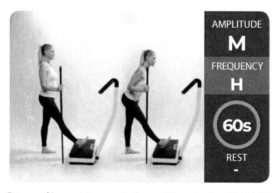

Standing Hamstring Stretch RIGHT

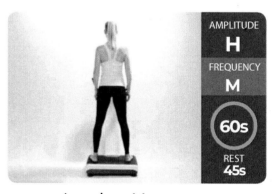

Lumbar Massage

Active Fitness Advanced

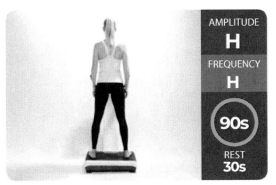

AMPLITUDE	H
FREQUENCY	H
90s	
REST	30s

Wide Stance

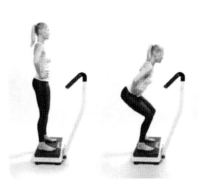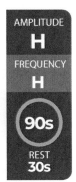

AMPLITUDE	H
FREQUENCY	H
90s	
REST	30s

Mini Squat

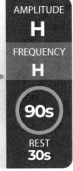

AMPLITUDE	H
FREQUENCY	H
90s	
REST	30s

Deep Squat

AMPLITUDE	H
FREQUENCY	H
60s	
REST	30s

Modified Push Up

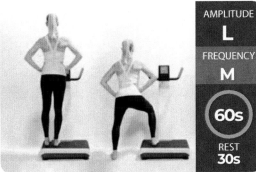

AMPLITUDE	L
FREQUENCY	M
60s	
REST	30s

Lateral Step Up LEFT

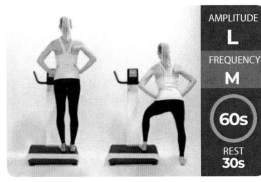

AMPLITUDE	L
FREQUENCY	M
60s	
REST	30s

Lateral Step Up RIGHT

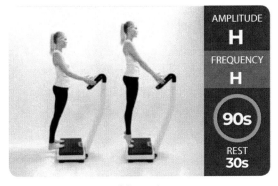

AMPLITUDE	H
FREQUENCY	H
90s	
REST	30s

Calf Raise

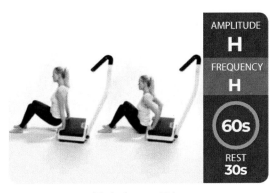

AMPLITUDE	H
FREQUENCY	H
60s	
REST	30s

Triceps Dip

Active Fitness Advanced

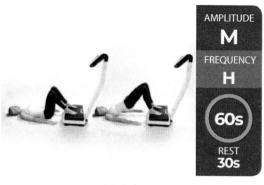

Bridge

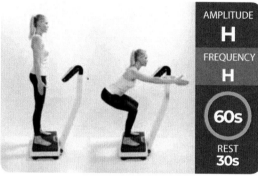

Plank with Extended Elbows

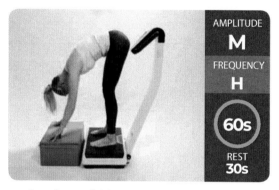

Deep Squat

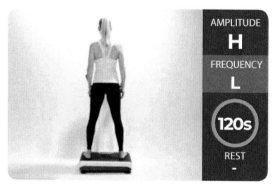

Assisted Hamstring Stretch

Lumbar Massage

Bone Building

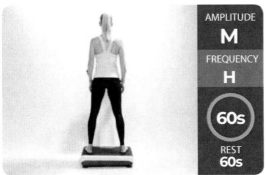
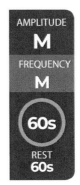

AMPLITUDE
M
FREQUENCY
H
60s
REST
60s

Wide Stance

AMPLITUDE
M
FREQUENCY
M
60s
REST
60s

Normal Stance

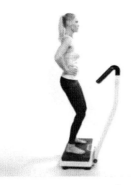
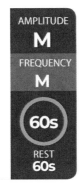

AMPLITUDE
M
FREQUENCY
M
60s
REST
60s

Normal Stance

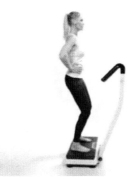
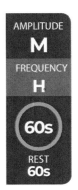

AMPLITUDE
M
FREQUENCY
H
60s
REST
60s

Normal Stance

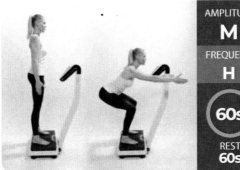
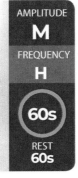

AMPLITUDE
M
FREQUENCY
H
60s
REST
60s

Deep Squat

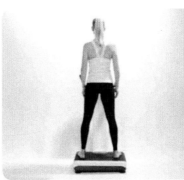
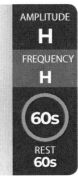

AMPLITUDE
H
FREQUENCY
H
60s
REST
60s

Lumbar Massage

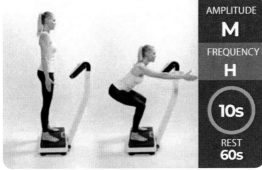
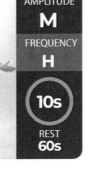

AMPLITUDE
M
FREQUENCY
H
10s
REST
60s

Deep Squat

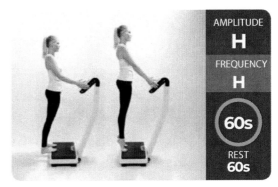

AMPLITUDE
H
FREQUENCY
H
60s
REST
60s

Calf Raise

Bone Building

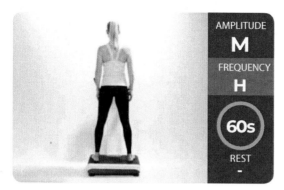

Lumbar Massage

Balance

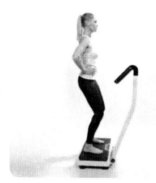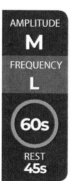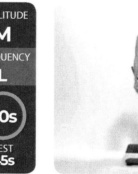

Normal Stance

Narrow Stance

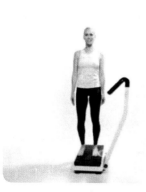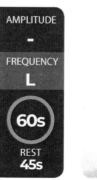

Wide Side Stance

Narrow Side Stance

Balance

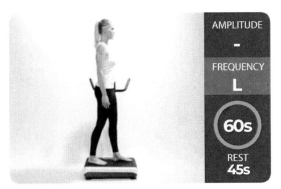

Tandem Side Stance

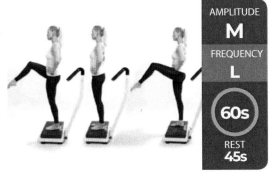

Alternating Knee Lift

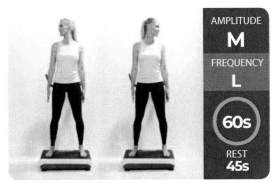

Wide Stance with Head Turn

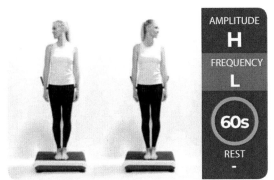

Narrow Stance with Head Turn

Balance Progression

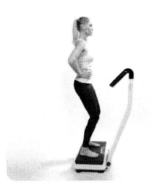

Normal Stance

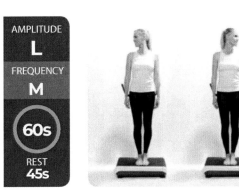

Narrow Stance with Head Turn

Balance Progression

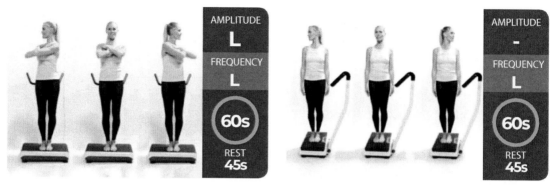

AMPLITUDE	AMPLITUDE
L	-
FREQUENCY	FREQUENCY
L	L
60s	60s
REST 45s	REST 45s

Narrow Stance with Rotation   Narrow Side Stance with Head Turn

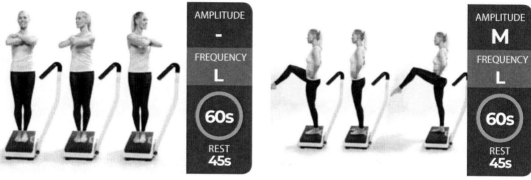

AMPLITUDE	AMPLITUDE
-	M
FREQUENCY	FREQUENCY
L	L
60s	60s
REST 45s	REST 45s

Narrow Side Stance with Rotation   Alternating Knee Lift

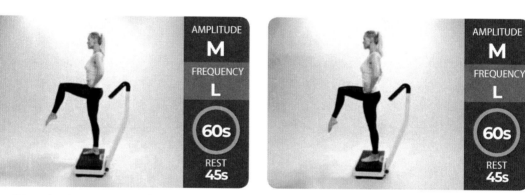

AMPLITUDE	AMPLITUDE
M	M
FREQUENCY	FREQUENCY
L	L
60s	60s
REST 45s	REST 45s

Single Leg Standing LEFT   Single Leg Standing RIGHT

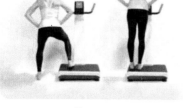

AMPLITUDE	AMPLITUDE
M	M
FREQUENCY	FREQUENCY
L	L
45s	45s
REST 45s	REST -

Step Up LEFT   Step Up RIGHT

Active Pelvic Floor

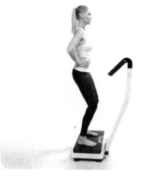

AMPLITUDE L
FREQUENCY M
60s
REST 45s

Normal Stance

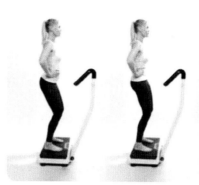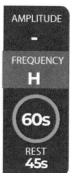

AMPLITUDE -
FREQUENCY H
60s
REST 45s

Pelvic Tilts

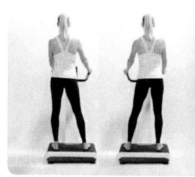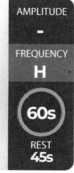

AMPLITUDE -
FREQUENCY H
60s
REST 45s

Standing Weight Shift

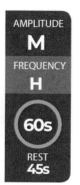

AMPLITUDE M
FREQUENCY H
60s
REST 45s

Mini Squat

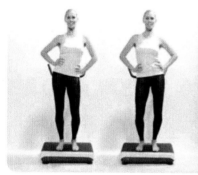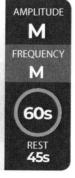

AMPLITUDE M
FREQUENCY M
60s
REST 45s

Hip Circles

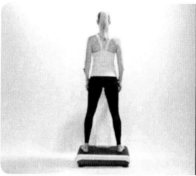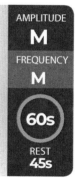

AMPLITUDE M
FREQUENCY M
60s
REST 45s

Wide Stance

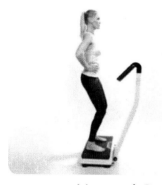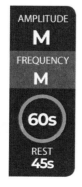

AMPLITUDE M
FREQUENCY M
60s
REST 45s

Normal Stance

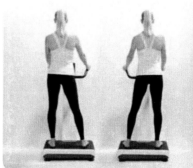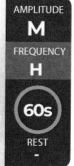

AMPLITUDE M
FREQUENCY H
60s
REST -

Standing Weight Shift

Active Flexibility

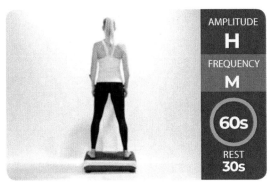

Wide Stance

AMPLITUDE **H**
FREQUENCY **M**
60s
REST **30s**

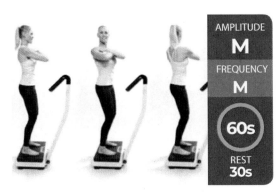

Lumbar Rotation

AMPLITUDE **M**
FREQUENCY **M**
60s
REST **30s**

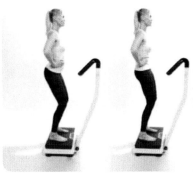

Pelvic Tilts

AMPLITUDE **M**
FREQUENCY **M**
60s
REST **30s**

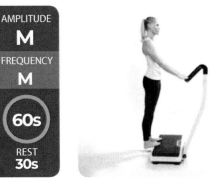

Calf Stretch

AMPLITUDE **H**
FREQUENCY **H**
60s
REST **30s**

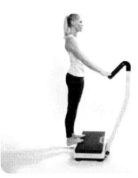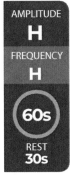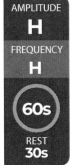

Calf Stretch

AMPLITUDE **H**
FREQUENCY **H**
60s
REST **30s**

Standing Hamstring Stretch LEFT

AMPLITUDE **M**
FREQUENCY **H**
60s
REST **30s**

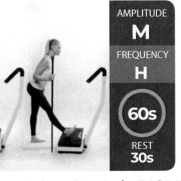

Standing Hamstring Stretch RIGHT

AMPLITUDE **M**
FREQUENCY **H**
60s
REST **30s**

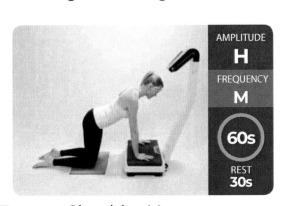

Shoulder Massage

AMPLITUDE **H**
FREQUENCY **M**
60s
REST **30s**

Active Flexibility

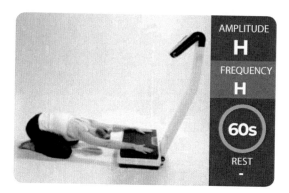

AMPLITUDE
H

FREQUENCY
H

60s

REST
-

Prayer Stretch

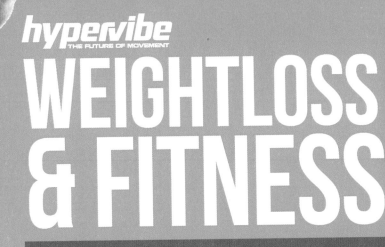

hypervibe
THE FUTURE OF MOVEMENT

WEIGHTLOSS & FITNESS

EXERCISE GUIDE

For people of all ages who want an effective way to lose weight, feel strong, and improve their energy levels.

GIO MINI

GIO

Fitness Introduction

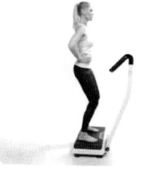

AMPLITUDE
M
FREQUENCY
H
45s
REST
45s

Normal Stance

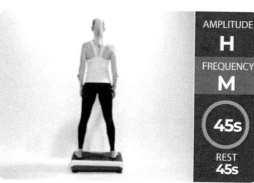

AMPLITUDE
H
FREQUENCY
M
45s
REST
45s

Wide Stance

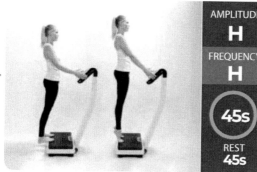

AMPLITUDE
H
FREQUENCY
H
45s
REST
45s

Calf Raise

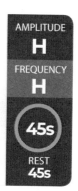

AMPLITUDE
H
FREQUENCY
H
45s
REST
45s

Mini Squat

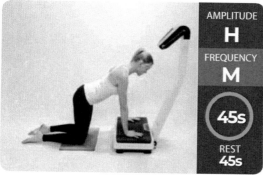

AMPLITUDE
H
FREQUENCY
M
45s
REST
45s

Shoulder Massage

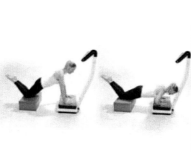

AMPLITUDE
H
FREQUENCY
L
45s
REST
45s

Modified Push Up

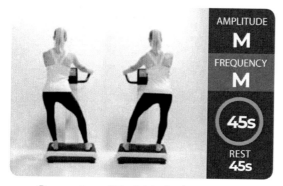

AMPLITUDE
M
FREQUENCY
M
45s
REST
45s

Squat with Weight Shift

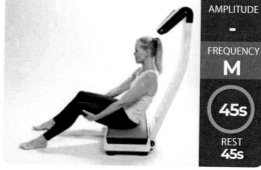

AMPLITUDE
-
FREQUENCY
M
45s
REST
45s

Seated Massage

Fitness Introduction

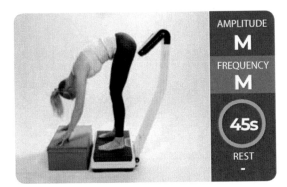

Assisted Hamstring Stretch

Total Body Fitness Beginner

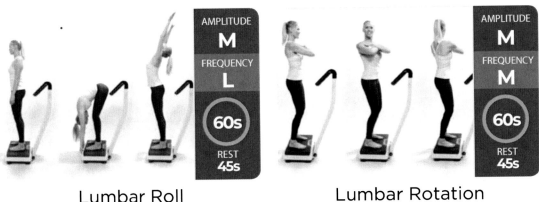

Lumbar Roll

Lumbar Rotation

Deep Squat

Push-Up

Total Body Fitness Beginner

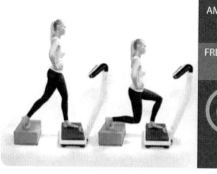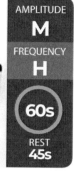

AMPLITUDE **M**
FREQUENCY **H**
60s
REST **45s**

Lunge LEFT

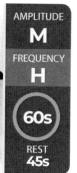

AMPLITUDE **M**
FREQUENCY **H**
60s
REST **45s**

Lunge RIGHT

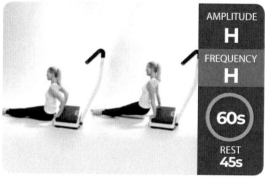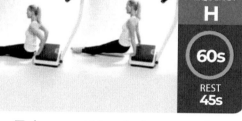

AMPLITUDE **H**
FREQUENCY **H**
60s
REST **45s**

Triceps Dip Advanced

AMPLITUDE **H**
FREQUENCY **H**
60s
REST **45s**

Plank with Extended Elbows

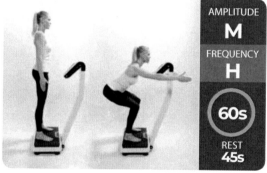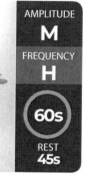

AMPLITUDE **M**
FREQUENCY **H**
60s
REST **45s**

Deep Squat

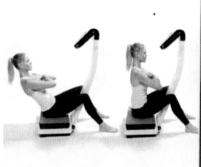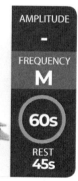

AMPLITUDE **-**
FREQUENCY **M**
60s
REST **45s**

Abdominal Crunch

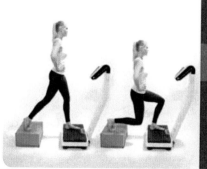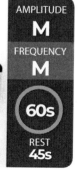

AMPLITUDE **M**
FREQUENCY **M**
60s
REST **45s**

Bridge

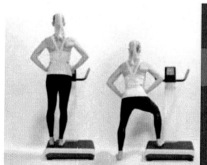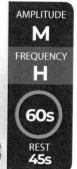

AMPLITUDE **M**
FREQUENCY **H**
60s
REST **45s**

Lateral Step Up

Total Body Fitness Beginner

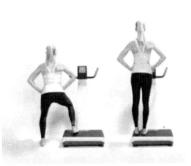 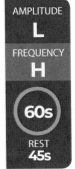

AMPLITUDE	L
FREQUENCY	H
60s	
REST	45s

Step Up LEFT

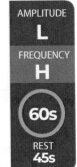

AMPLITUDE	L
FREQUENCY	H
60s	
REST	45s

Step Up RIGHT

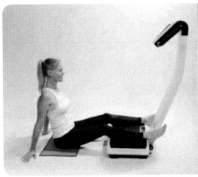 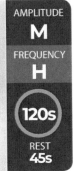

AMPLITUDE	M
FREQUENCY	H
120s	
REST	45s

Calf Massage

AMPLITUDE	M
FREQUENCY	H
120s	
REST	45s

Hamstring Massage

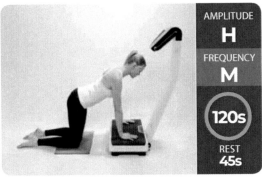 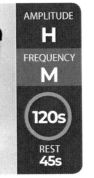

AMPLITUDE	H
FREQUENCY	M
120s	
REST	45s

Shoulder Massage

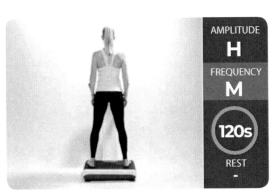

AMPLITUDE	H
FREQUENCY	M
120s	
REST	-

Wide Stance

Total Body Fitness Intermediate

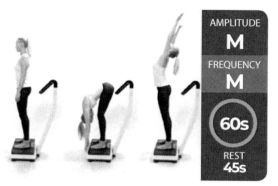

Lumbar Roll

AMPLITUDE **M**
FREQUENCY **M**
60s
REST **45s**

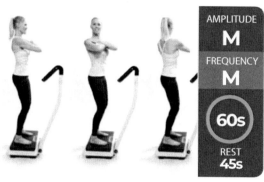

Lumbar Rotation

AMPLITUDE **M**
FREQUENCY **M**
60s
REST **45s**

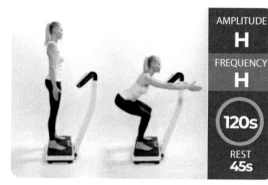

Deep Squat

AMPLITUDE **H**
FREQUENCY **H**
120s
REST **45s**

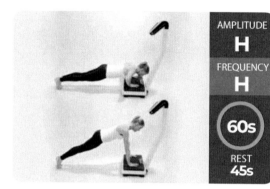

Push-Up

AMPLITUDE **H**
FREQUENCY **H**
60s
REST **45s**

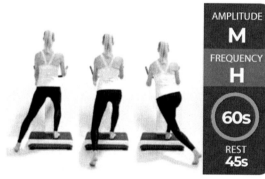

3 Way Lunge LEFT

AMPLITUDE **M**
FREQUENCY **H**
60s
REST **45s**

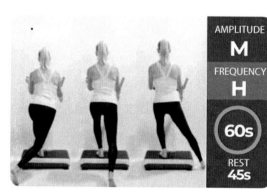

3 Way Lunge RIGHT

AMPLITUDE **M**
FREQUENCY **H**
60s
REST **45s**

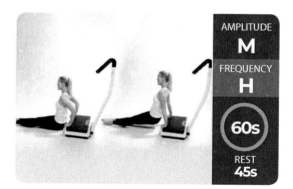

Triceps Dip Advanced

AMPLITUDE **M**
FREQUENCY **H**
60s
REST **45s**

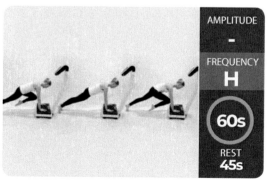

Plank with Mountain Climber

AMPLITUDE **-**
FREQUENCY **H**
60s
REST **45s**

Total Body Fitness Intermediate

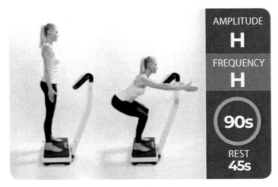

AMPLITUDE H
FREQUENCY H
90s
REST 45s

Deep Squat

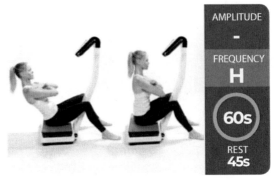

AMPLITUDE -
FREQUENCY H
60s
REST 45s

Abdominal Crunch

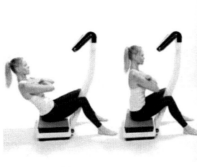

AMPLITUDE -
FREQUENCY H
60s
REST 45s

Abdominal Crunch

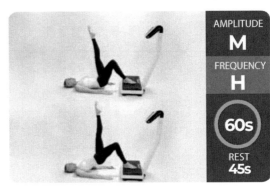

AMPLITUDE M
FREQUENCY H
60s
REST 45s

Single Leg Bridge LEFT

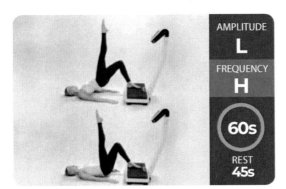

AMPLITUDE L
FREQUENCY H
60s
REST 45s

Single Leg Bridge RIGHT

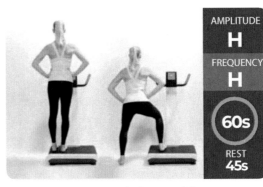

AMPLITUDE H
FREQUENCY H
60s
REST 45s

Lateral Step Up

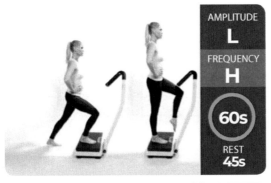

AMPLITUDE L
FREQUENCY H
60s
REST 45s

Step Up with Knee Lift LEFT

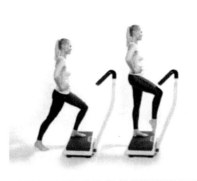

AMPLITUDE L
FREQUENCY H
60s
REST 45s

Step Up with Knee Lift RIGHT

Total Body Fitness Intermediate

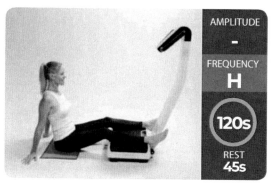

Calf Massage

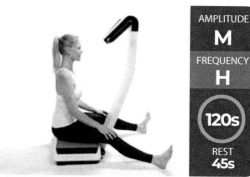

Hamstring Massage

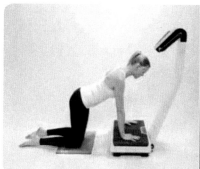

Shoulder Massage

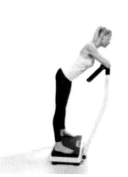

Lumbar Massage

Total Body Fitness Advanced

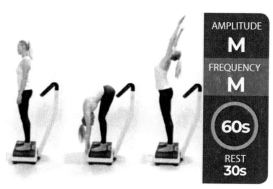

Lumbar Roll

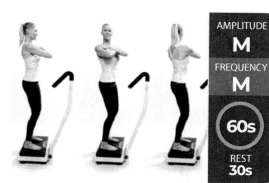

Lumbar Rotation

Total Body Fitness Advanced

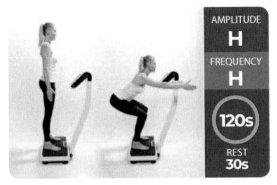

Deep Squat

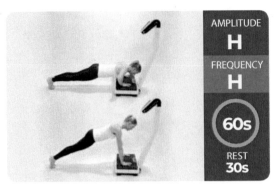

Push-Up

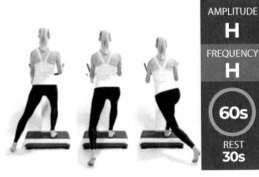

3 Way Lunge LEFT

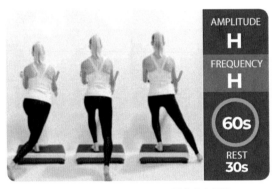

3 Way Lunge RIGHT

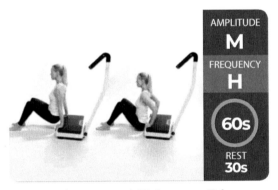

Advanced Triceps Dip

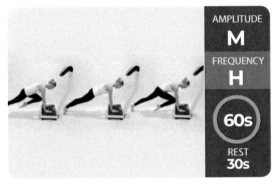

Plank with Mountain Climber

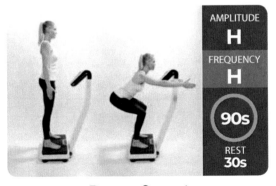

Deep Squat

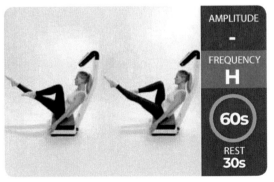

Advanced Abdominals

Total Body Fitness Advanced

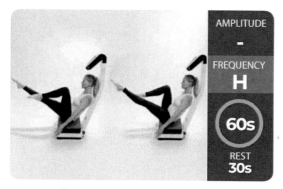

Advanced Abdominals

AMPLITUDE -
FREQUENCY H
60s
REST 30s

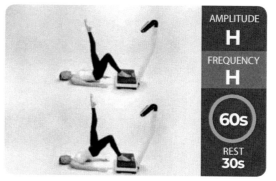

Single Leg Bridge LEFT

AMPLITUDE H
FREQUENCY H
60s
REST 30s

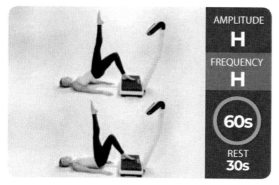

Single Leg Bridge RIGHT

AMPLITUDE H
FREQUENCY H
60s
REST 30s

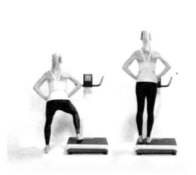

Lateral Step Up

AMPLITUDE L
FREQUENCY H
60s
REST 30s

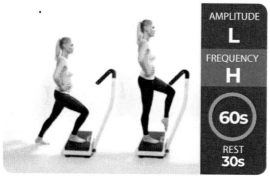

Step Up with Knee Lift LEFT

AMPLITUDE L
FREQUENCY H
60s
REST 30s

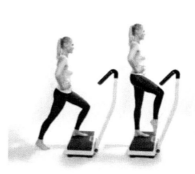

Step Up with Knee Lift RIGHT

AMPLITUDE M
FREQUENCY H
60s
REST 30s

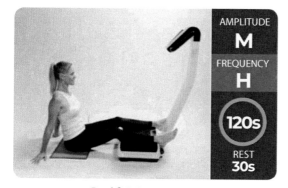

Calf Massage

AMPLITUDE M
FREQUENCY H
120s
REST 30s

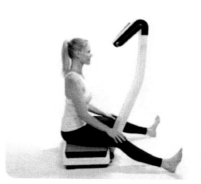

Hamstring Massage

AMPLITUDE M
FREQUENCY H
120s
REST 30s

Total Body Fitness Advanced

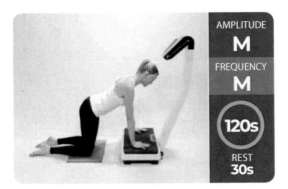

Shoulder Massage

AMPLITUDE **M**
FREQUENCY **M**
120s
REST **30s**

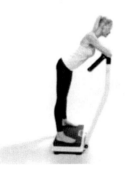

Lumbar Massage

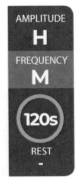

AMPLITUDE **H**
FREQUENCY **M**
120s
REST **-**

Core Basic

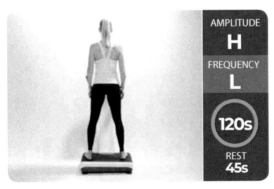

Wide Stance

AMPLITUDE **H**
FREQUENCY **L**
120s
REST **45s**

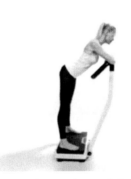

Lumbar Massage

AMPLITUDE **M**
FREQUENCY **M**
90s
REST **45s**

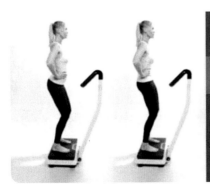

Pelvic Tilts

AMPLITUDE **M**
FREQUENCY **M**
60s
REST **45s**

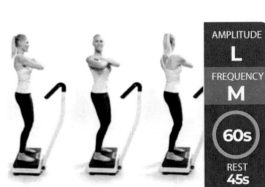

Lumbar Rotation

AMPLITUDE **L**
FREQUENCY **M**
60s
REST **45s**

Core Basic

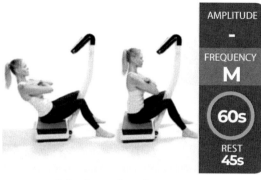

Abdominal Crunch

AMPLITUDE
-
FREQUENCY
M
60s
REST
45s

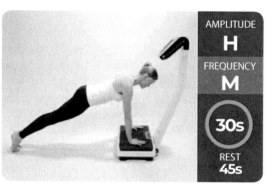

Plank with Extended Elbows

AMPLITUDE
H
FREQUENCY
M
30s
REST
45s

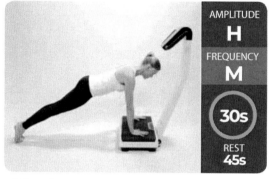

Plank with Extended Elbows

AMPLITUDE
H
FREQUENCY
M
30s
REST
45s

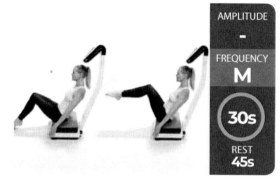

Abdominal Knee Lift

AMPLITUDE
-
FREQUENCY
M
30s
REST
45s

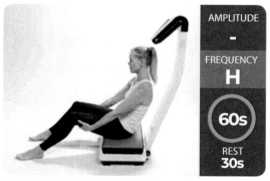

Seated Massage

AMPLITUDE
-
FREQUENCY
H
60s
REST
30s

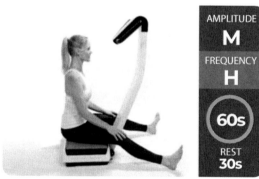

Hamstring Massage

AMPLITUDE
M
FREQUENCY
H
60s
REST
30s

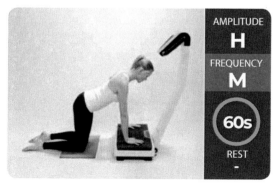

Shoulder Massage

AMPLITUDE
H
FREQUENCY
M
60s
REST
-

Core Intermediate

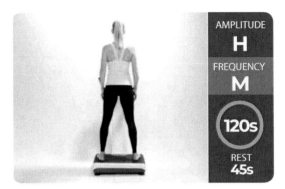

AMPLITUDE
H
FREQUENCY
M
120s
REST
45s

Wide Stance

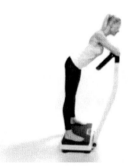

AMPLITUDE
M
FREQUENCY
M
90s
REST
45s

Lumbar Massage

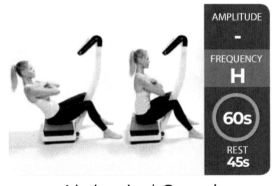

AMPLITUDE
M
FREQUENCY
H
60s
REST
45s

Lumbar Rotation

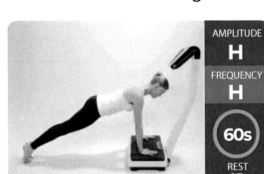

AMPLITUDE
H
FREQUENCY
H
60s
REST
45s

Plank with Extended Elbows

AMPLITUDE
-
FREQUENCY
H
60s
REST
45s

Abdominal Crunch

AMPLITUDE
-
FREQUENCY
H
60s
REST
45s

Abdominal Knee Lift

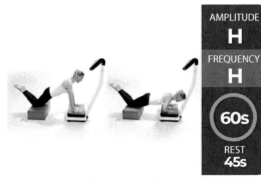

AMPLITUDE
H
FREQUENCY
H
60s
REST
45s

Modified Push-up

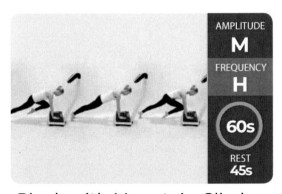

AMPLITUDE
M
FREQUENCY
H
60s
REST
45s

Plank with Mountain Climber

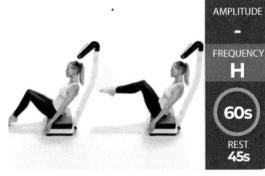

Core Intermediate

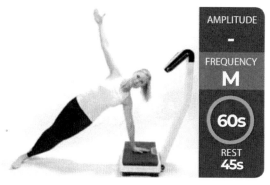

Side Plank LEFT

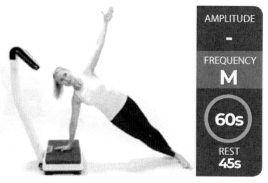

Side Plank RIGHT

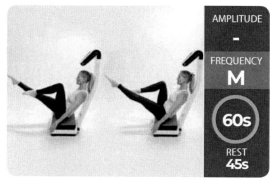

Advanced Abdominals

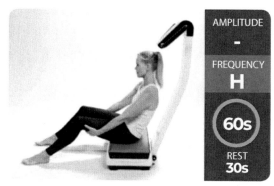

Seated Massage

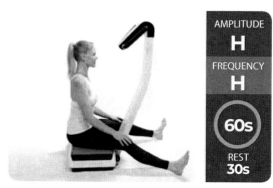

Hamstring Massage

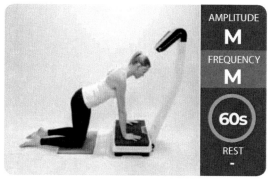

Shoulder Massage

Core Advanced

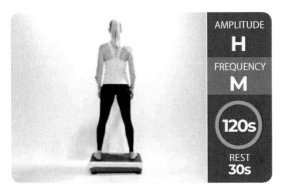

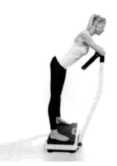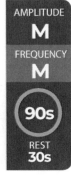

AMPLITUDE	H
FREQUENCY	M
120s	
REST	30s

Wide Stance

AMPLITUDE	M
FREQUENCY	M
90s	
REST	30s

Lumbar Massage

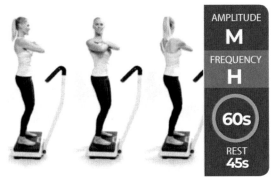

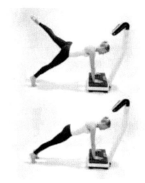

AMPLITUDE	M
FREQUENCY	H
60s	
REST	45s

Lumbar Rotation

AMPLITUDE	H
FREQUENCY	H
60s	
REST	30s

Plank with Hip Extension

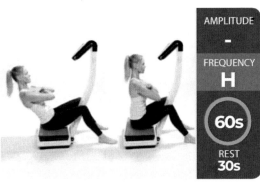

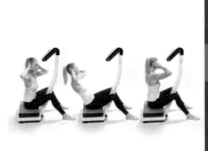

AMPLITUDE	-
FREQUENCY	H
60s	
REST	30s

Abdominal Crunch

AMPLITUDE	-
FREQUENCY	H
60s	
REST	30s

Torso Twist

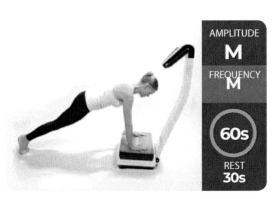

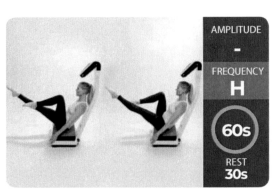

AMPLITUDE	M
FREQUENCY	M
60s	
REST	30s

Standard Plank

AMPLITUDE	-
FREQUENCY	H
60s	
REST	30s

Advanced Abdominals

Core Advanced

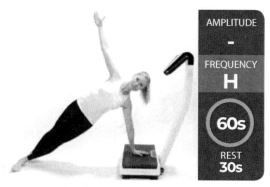

Side Plank LEFT

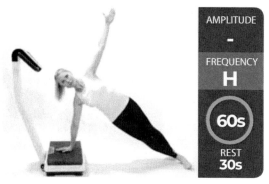

Side Plank RIGHT

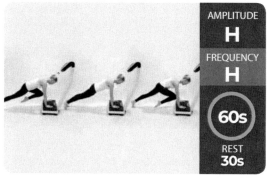

Plank with Mountain Climber

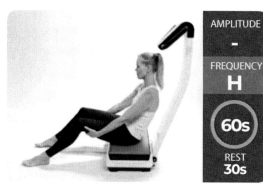

Seated Massage

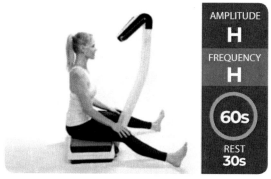

Hamstring Massage

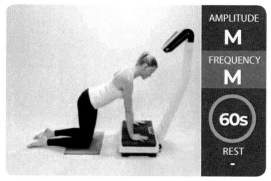

Shoulder Massage

Flexibility

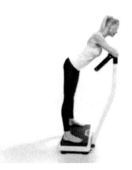

AMPLITUDE	H
FREQUENCY	M
90s	
REST	30s

Lumbar Massage

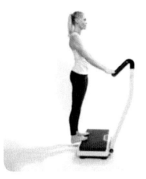

AMPLITUDE	L
FREQUENCY	H
90s	
REST	30s

Standing Hamstring Stretch

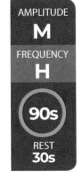

AMPLITUDE	M
FREQUENCY	H
90s	
REST	30s

Calf Stretch

AMPLITUDE	M
FREQUENCY	H
90s	
REST	30s

Calf Stretch

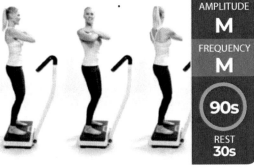

AMPLITUDE	M
FREQUENCY	M
90s	
REST	30s

Lumbar Rotation

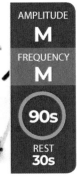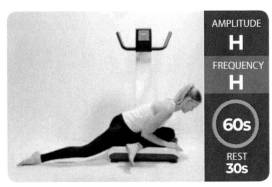

AMPLITUDE	H
FREQUENCY	H
60s	
REST	30s

Pigeon Stretch LEFT

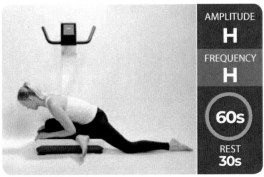

AMPLITUDE	H
FREQUENCY	H
60s	
REST	30s

Pigeon Stretch RIGHT

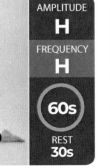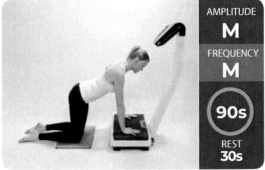

AMPLITUDE	M
FREQUENCY	M
90s	
REST	30s

Shoulder Massage

Flexibility

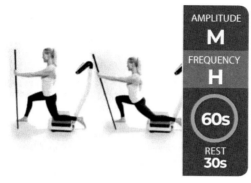

Assisted Hip Flexor Stretch LEFT

Assisted Hip Flexor Stretch RIGHT

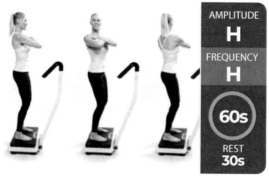

Lumbar Rotation

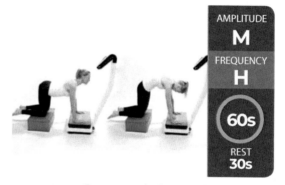

Cat and Camel

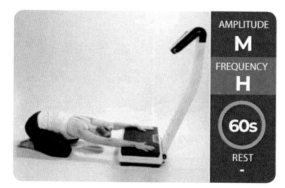

Prayer Stretch

Tabata Beginner

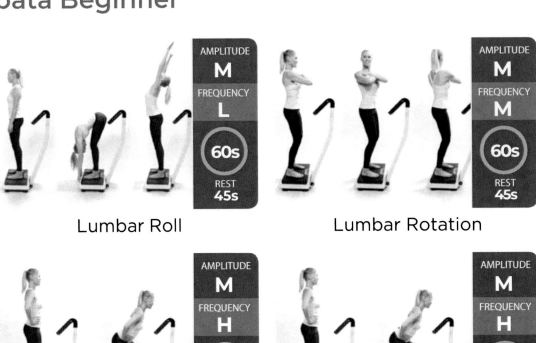

Lumbar Roll

Lumbar Rotation

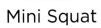

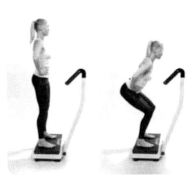

Mini Squat

Mini Squat

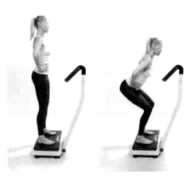

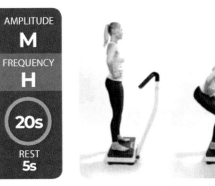

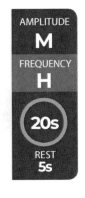

Mini Squat

Mini Squat

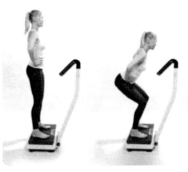

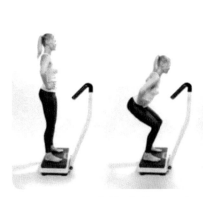

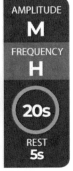

Mini Squat

Mini Squat

Tabata Beginner

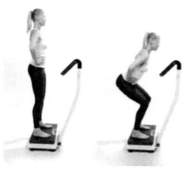 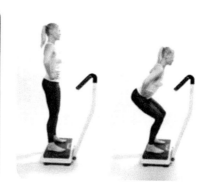 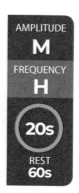

Mini Squat

Mini Squat

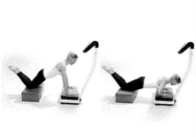 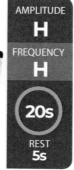 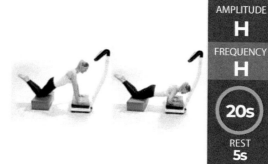

Modified Push-up

Modified Push-up

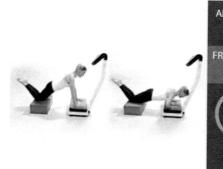 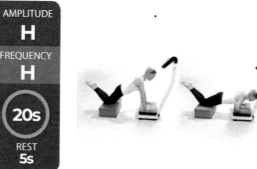

Modified Push-up

Modified Push-up

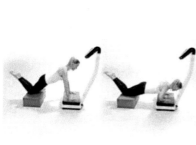 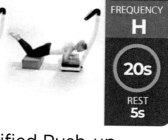 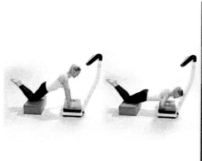 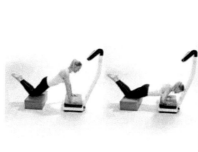

Modified Push-up

Modified Push-up

Tabata Beginner

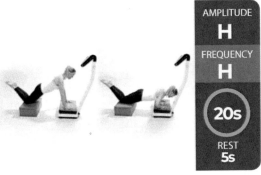

Modified Push-up

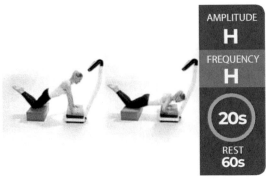

Modified Push-up

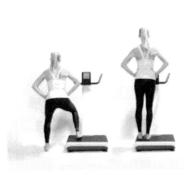

Step Up LEFT

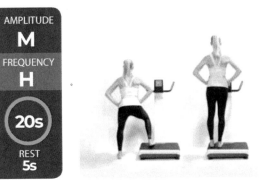

Step Up LEFT

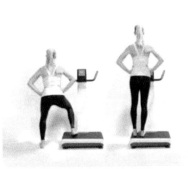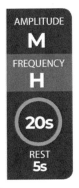

Step Up LEFT

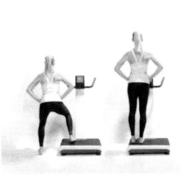

Step Up LEFT

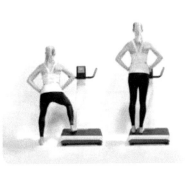

Step Up LEFT

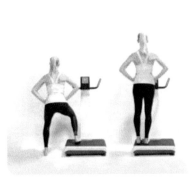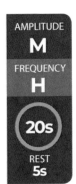

Step Up LEFT

Tabata Beginner

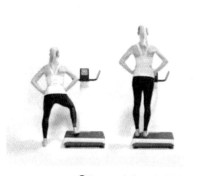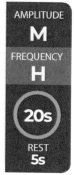

Step Up LEFT

AMPLITUDE **M** FREQUENCY **H** 20s REST 5s

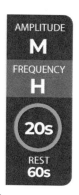

Step Up LEFT

AMPLITUDE **M** FREQUENCY **H** 20s REST 60s

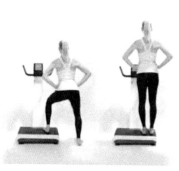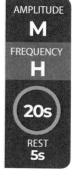

Step Up RIGHT

AMPLITUDE **M** FREQUENCY **H** 20s REST 5s

Step Up RIGHT

AMPLITUDE **M** FREQUENCY **H** 20s REST 5s

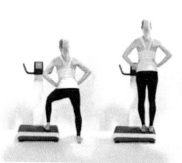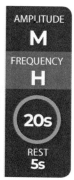

Step Up RIGHT

AMPLITUDE **M** FREQUENCY **H** 20s REST 5s

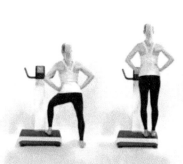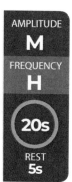

Step Up RIGHT

AMPLITUDE **M** FREQUENCY **H** 20s REST 5s

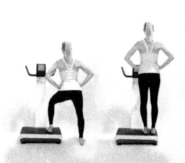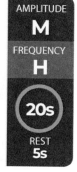

Step Up RIGHT

AMPLITUDE **M** FREQUENCY **H** 20s REST 5s

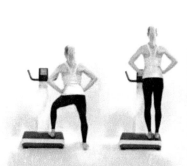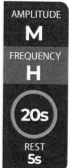

Step Up RIGHT

AMPLITUDE **M** FREQUENCY **H** 20s REST 5s

Tabata Beginner

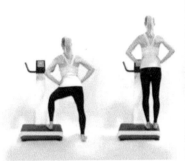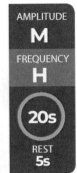

AMPLITUDE
M
FREQUENCY
H
20s
REST
5s

Step Up RIGHT

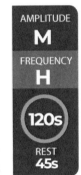

AMPLITUDE
M
FREQUENCY
H
20s
REST
5s

Step Up RIGHT

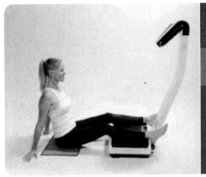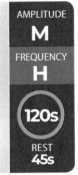

AMPLITUDE
M
FREQUENCY
H
120s
REST
45s

Calf Massage

AMPLITUDE
M
FREQUENCY
H
120s
REST
45s

Hamstring Massage

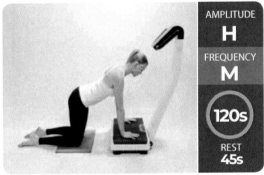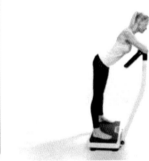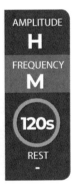

AMPLITUDE
H
FREQUENCY
M
120s
REST
45s

Shoulder Massage

AMPLITUDE
H
FREQUENCY
M
120s
REST
-

Lumbar Massage

Tabata Intermediate

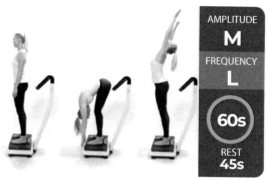

AMPLITUDE
M
FREQUENCY
L
60s
REST
45s

Lumbar Roll

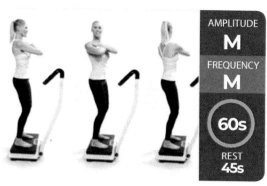

AMPLITUDE
M
FREQUENCY
M
60s
REST
45s

Lumbar Rotation

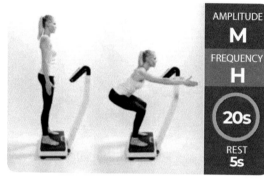

AMPLITUDE
M
FREQUENCY
H
20s
REST
5s

Deep Squat

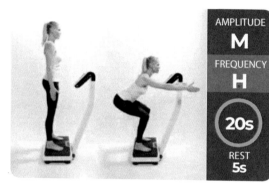

AMPLITUDE
M
FREQUENCY
H
20s
REST
5s

Deep Squat

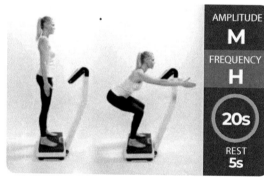

AMPLITUDE
M
FREQUENCY
H
20s
REST
5s

Deep Squat

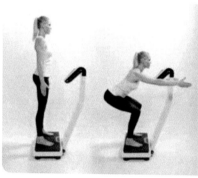

AMPLITUDE
M
FREQUENCY
H
20s
REST
5s

Deep Squat

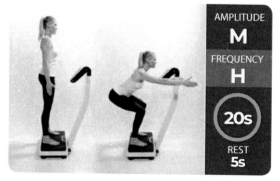

AMPLITUDE
M
FREQUENCY
H
20s
REST
5s

Deep Squat

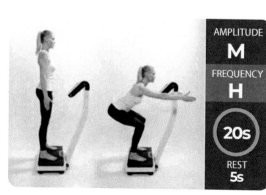

AMPLITUDE
M
FREQUENCY
H
20s
REST
5s

Deep Squat

Tabata Intermediate

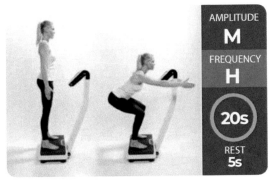

Deep Squat

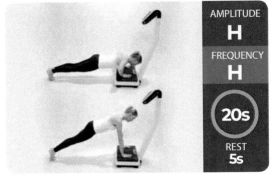

Deep Squat

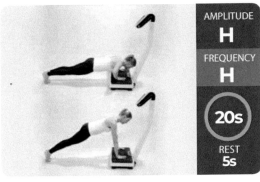

Push Up

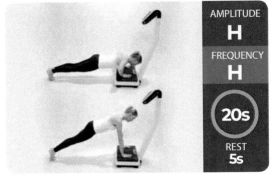

Push Up

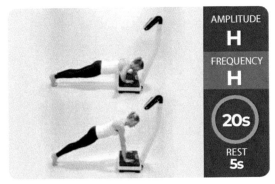

Push Up

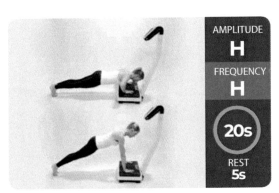

Push Up

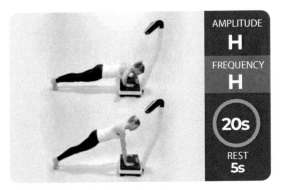

Push Up

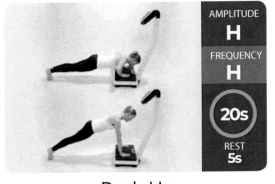

Push Up

Tabata Intermediate

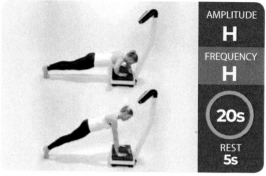

Push Up

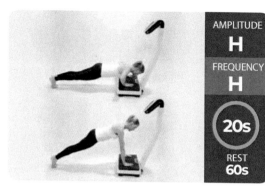

Push Up

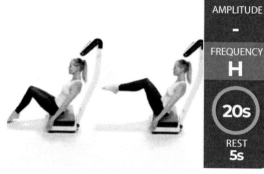

Abdominal Knee Lift

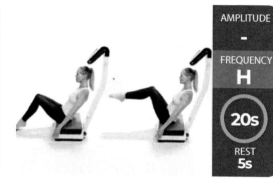

Abdominal Knee Lift

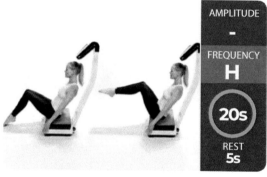

Abdominal Knee Lift

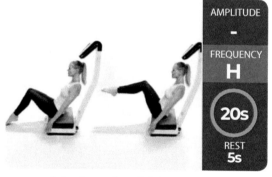

Abdominal Knee Lift

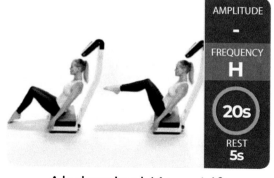

Abdominal Knee Lift

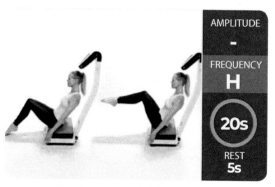

Abdominal Knee Lift

Tabata Intermediate

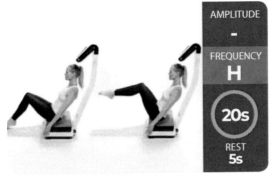

Abdominal Knee Lift

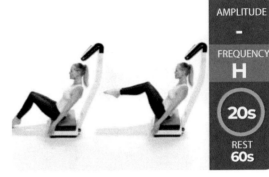

Abdominal Knee Lift

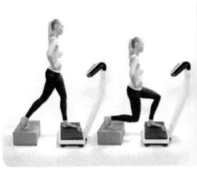

Lunge LEFT

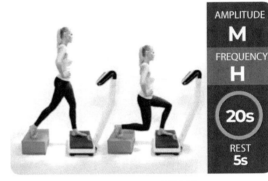

Lunge LEFT

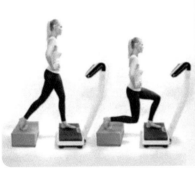

Lunge LEFT

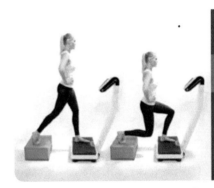

Lunge LEFT

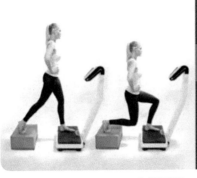

Lunge LEFT

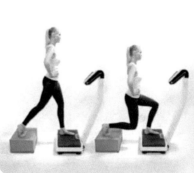
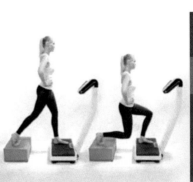

Lunge LEFT

Tabata Intermediate

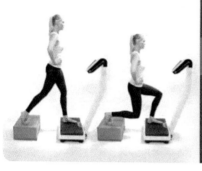 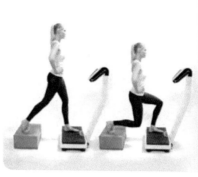 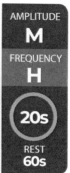

Lunge LEFT

Lunge LEFT

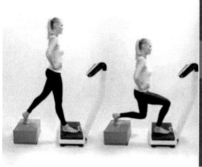 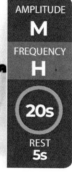

Lunge RIGHT

Lunge RIGHT

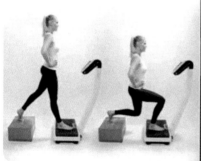 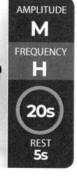 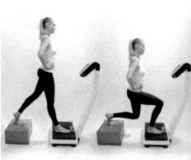 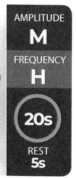

Lunge RIGHT

Lunge RIGHT

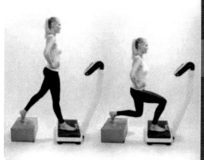 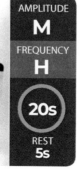 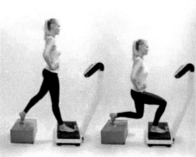 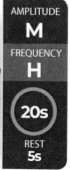

Lunge RIGHT

Lunge RIGHT

Tabata Intermediate

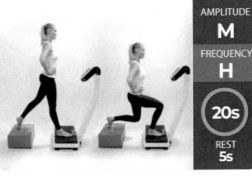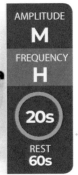

Lunge RIGHT

Lunge RIGHT

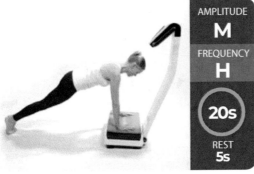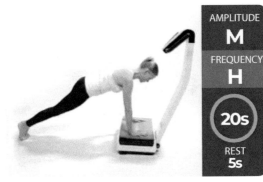

Standard Plank

Standard Plank

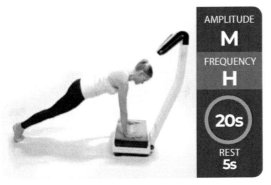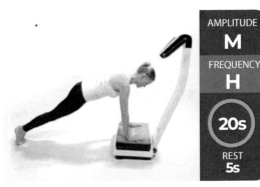

Standard Plank

Standard Plank

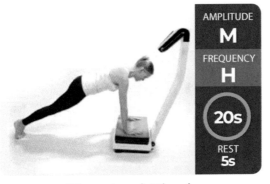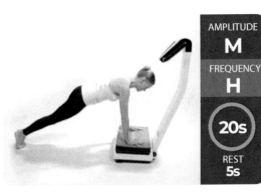

Standard Plank

Standard Plank

Tabata Intermediate

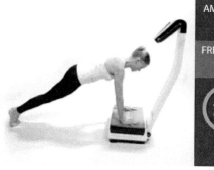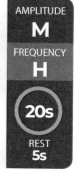

AMPLITUDE **M**
FREQUENCY **H**
20s
REST **5s**

Standard Plank

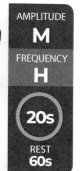

AMPLITUDE **M**
FREQUENCY **H**
20s
REST **60s**

Standard Plank

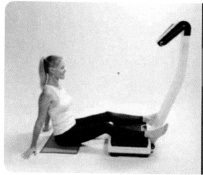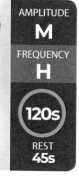

AMPLITUDE **M**
FREQUENCY **H**
120s
REST **45s**

Calf Massage

AMPLITUDE **M**
FREQUENCY **H**
120s
REST **45s**

Hamstring Massage

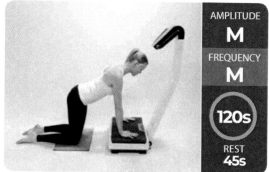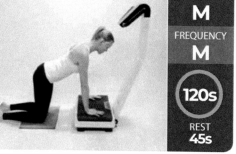

AMPLITUDE **M**
FREQUENCY **M**
120s
REST **45s**

Shoulder Massage

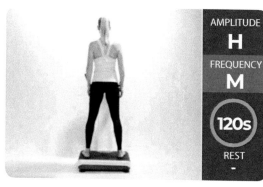

AMPLITUDE **H**
FREQUENCY **M**
120s
REST **-**

Lumbar Massage

Tabata Advanced

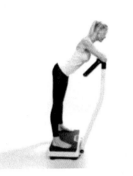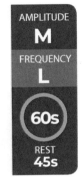

AMPLITUDE
M
FREQUENCY
L
60s
REST
45s

Lumbar Massage

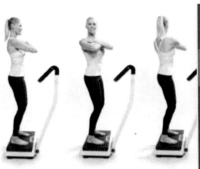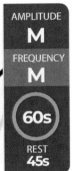

AMPLITUDE
M
FREQUENCY
M
60s
REST
45s

Lumbar Rotation

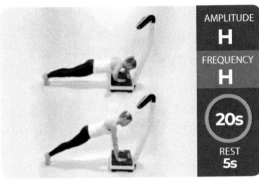

AMPLITUDE
H
FREQUENCY
H
20s
REST
5s

Push Up

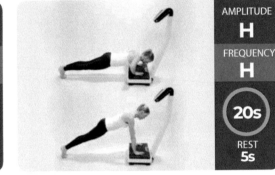

AMPLITUDE
H
FREQUENCY
H
20s
REST
5s

Push Up

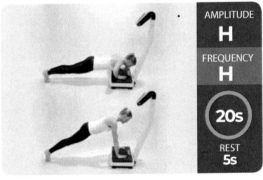

AMPLITUDE
H
FREQUENCY
H
20s
REST
5s

Push Up

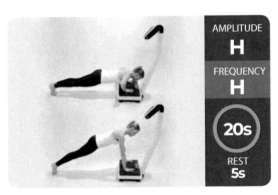

AMPLITUDE
H
FREQUENCY
H
20s
REST
5s

Push Up

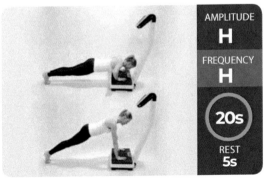

AMPLITUDE
H
FREQUENCY
H
20s
REST
5s

Push Up

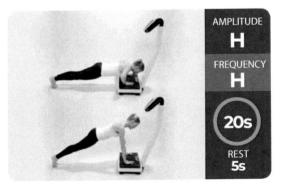

AMPLITUDE
H
FREQUENCY
H
20s
REST
5s

Push Up

Tabata Advanced

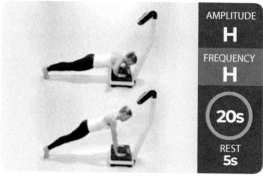

Push Up

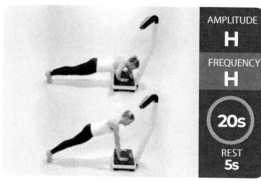

Push Up

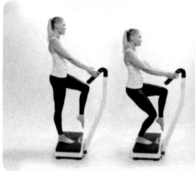

Single Leg Squat LEFT

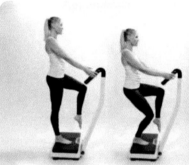

Single Leg Squat LEFT

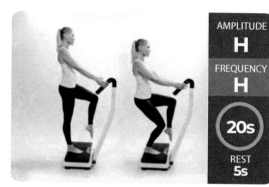

Single Leg Squat LEFT

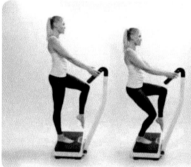

Single Leg Squat LEFT

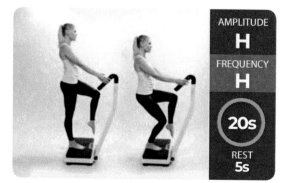

Single Leg Squat LEFT

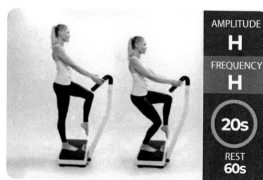

Single Leg Squat LEFT

Tabata Advanced

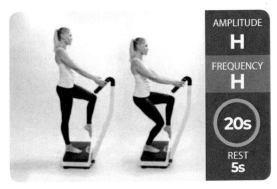

Single Leg Squat LEFT

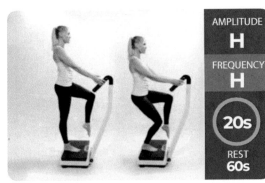

Single Leg Squat LEFT

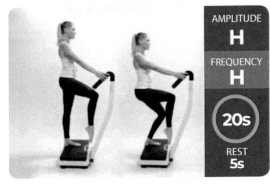

Single Leg Squat RIGHT

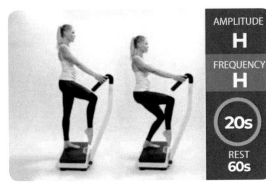

Single Leg Squat RIGHT

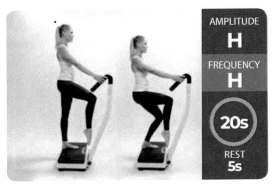

Single Leg Squat RIGHT

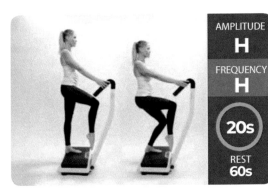

Single Leg Squat RIGHT

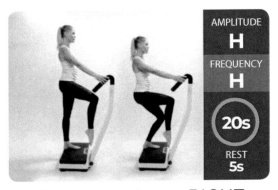

Single Leg Squat RIGHT

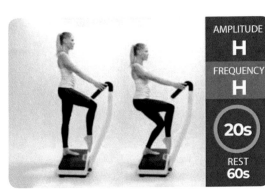

Single Leg Squat RIGHT

Tabata Advanced

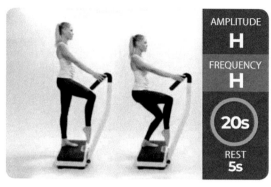

Single Leg Squat RIGHT

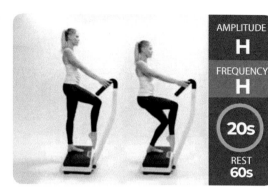

Single Leg Squat RIGHT

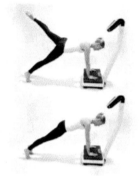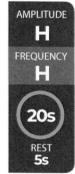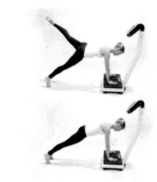

Plank with Hip Extension

Plank with Hip Extension

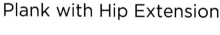

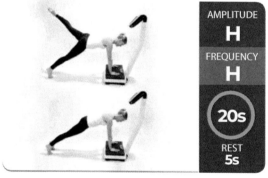

Plank with Hip Extension

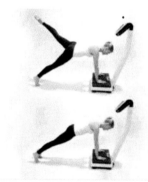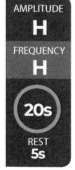

Plank with Hip Extension

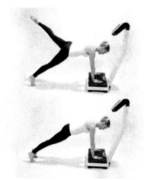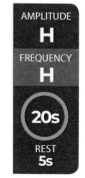

Plank with Hip Extension

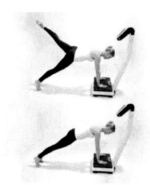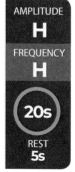

Plank with Hip Extension

Tabata Advanced

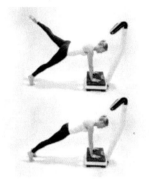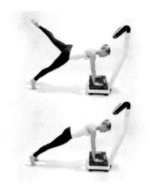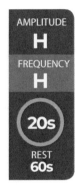

Plank with Hip Extension   Plank with Hip Extension

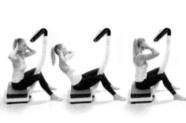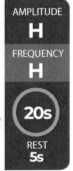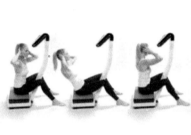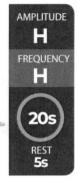

Torso Twist   Torso Twist

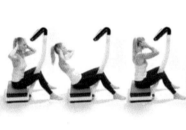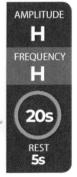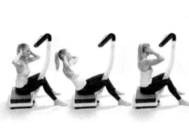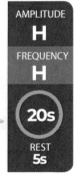

Torso Twist   Torso Twist

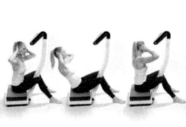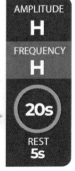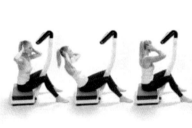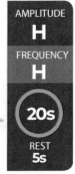

Torso Twist   Torso Twist

Tabata Advanced

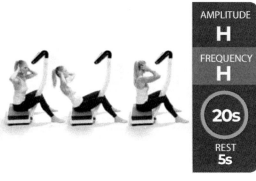
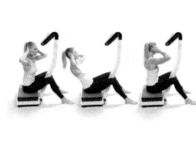
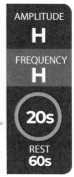

Torso Twist

Torso Twist

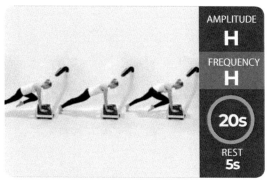

Plank with Mountain Climber

Plank with Mountain Climber

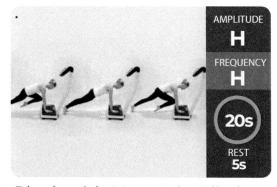

Plank with Mountain Climber

Plank with Mountain Climber

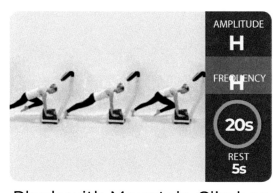
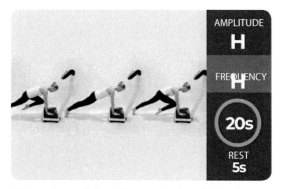

Plank with Mountain Climber

Plank with Mountain Climber

Tabata Advanced

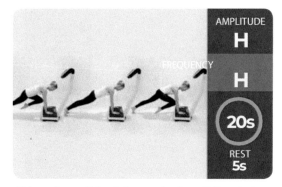

Plank with Mountain Climber

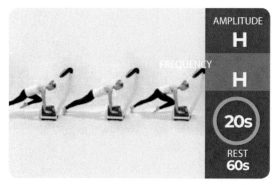

Plank with Mountain Climber

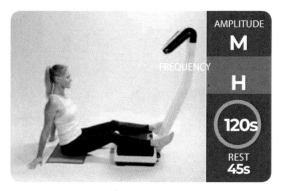

Calf Massage

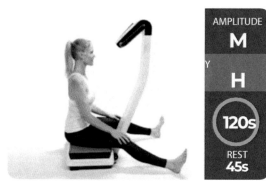

Hamstring Massage

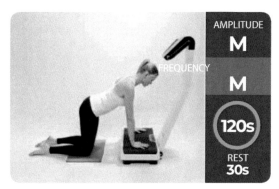

Shoulder Massage

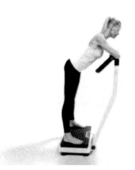

Lumbar Massage

hypervibe
THE FUTURE OF MOVEMENT

WOMEN'S HEALTH & FITNESS

EXERCISE GUIDE

For women who want a firmer figure, a more youthful appearance and regain their pre-pregnancy body.

Trim, Tight & Toned 1

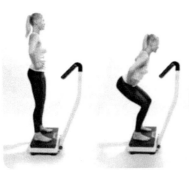

AMPLITUDE **H**
FREQUENCY **H**
60s
REST **45s**

Mini Squat

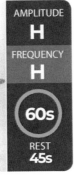

AMPLITUDE **H**
FREQUENCY **H**
30s
REST **30s**

Calf Raise

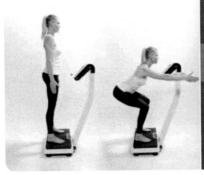

AMPLITUDE **H**
FREQUENCY **H**
60s
REST **45s**

Deep Squat

AMPLITUDE **M**
FREQUENCY **H**
30s
REST **45s**

Bridge

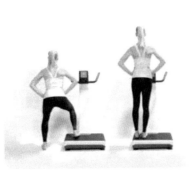

AMPLITUDE **L**
FREQUENCY **H**
30s
REST **45s**

Step Up LEFT

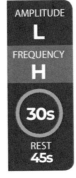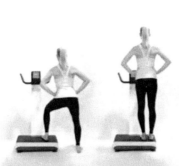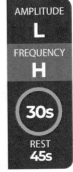

AMPLITUDE **L**
FREQUENCY **H**
30s
REST **45s**

Step Up RIGHT

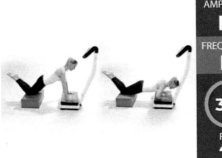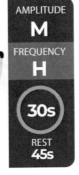

AMPLITUDE **M**
FREQUENCY **H**
30s
REST **45s**

Modified Pushup

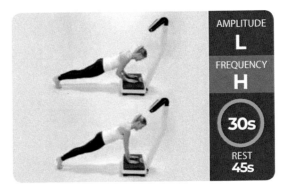

AMPLITUDE **L**
FREQUENCY **H**
30s
REST **45s**

Narrow Hands Pushup

Trim, Tight & Toned 1

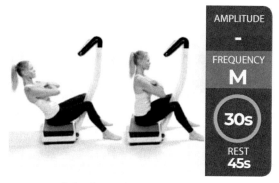

Abdominal Crunch

AMPLITUDE -
FREQUENCY M
30s
REST 45s

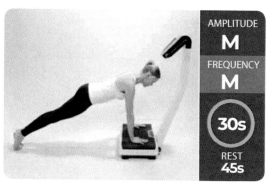

Plank with Extended Elbows

AMPLITUDE M
FREQUENCY M
30s
REST 45s

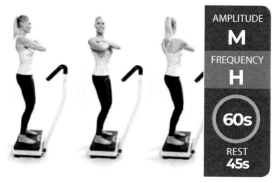

Lumbar Rotation

AMPLITUDE M
FREQUENCY H
60s
REST 45s

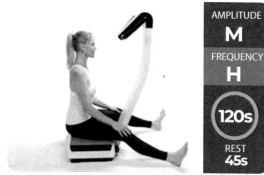

Hamstring Massage

AMPLITUDE M
FREQUENCY H
120s
REST 45s

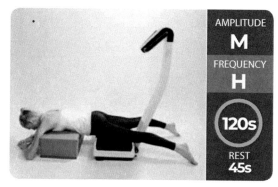

Quadriceps Massage

AMPLITUDE M
FREQUENCY H
120s
REST 45s

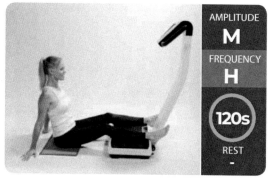

Calf Massage

AMPLITUDE M
FREQUENCY H
120s
REST -

Trim, Tight & Toned 2

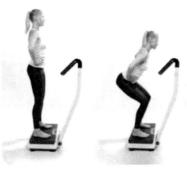

AMPLITUDE **H**
FREQUENCY **H**
60s
REST **45s**

Mini Squat

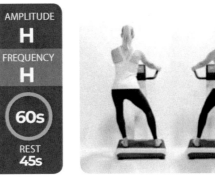

AMPLITUDE **H**
FREQUENCY **H**
60s
REST **45s**

Squat with Weight Shift

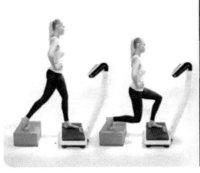

AMPLITUDE **H**
FREQUENCY **H**
60s
REST **45s**

Lunge LEFT

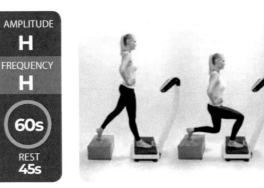

AMPLITUDE **H**
FREQUENCY **H**
60s
REST **45s**

Lunge RIGHT

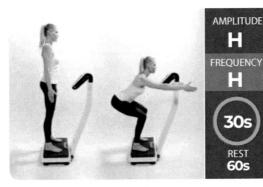

AMPLITUDE **H**
FREQUENCY **H**
30s
REST **60s**

Deep Squat

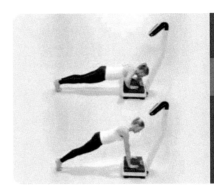

AMPLITUDE **H**
FREQUENCY **H**
60s
REST **45s**

Pushup

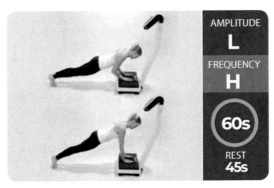

AMPLITUDE **L**
FREQUENCY **H**
60s
REST **45s**

Narrow Hands Pushup

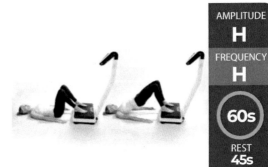

AMPLITUDE **H**
FREQUENCY **H**
60s
REST **45s**

Bridge

Trim, Tight & Toned 2

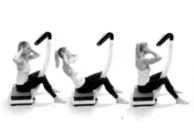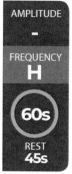

AMPLITUDE -
FREQUENCY H
60s
REST 45s

Torso Twist

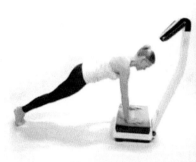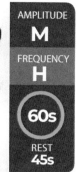

AMPLITUDE M
FREQUENCY H
60s
REST 45s

Standard Plank

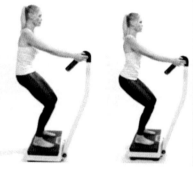

AMPLITUDE H
FREQUENCY H
60s
REST 45s

Squat with Pelvic Tilt

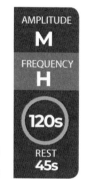

AMPLITUDE M
FREQUENCY H
120s
REST 45s

Hamstring Massage

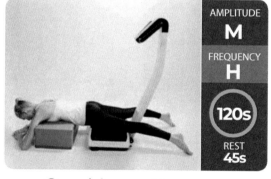

AMPLITUDE M
FREQUENCY H
120s
REST 45s

Quadriceps Massage

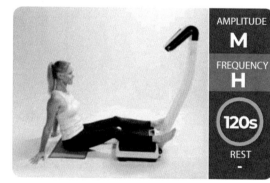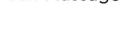

AMPLITUDE M
FREQUENCY H
120s
REST -

Calf Massage

Trim, Tight & Toned 3

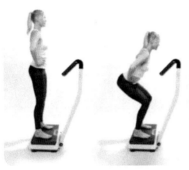

AMPLITUDE **H**
FREQUENCY **H**
120s
REST **30s**

Mini Squat

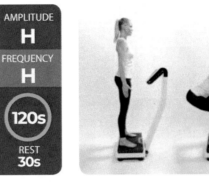

AMPLITUDE **H**
FREQUENCY **H**
90s
REST **30s**

Deep Squat

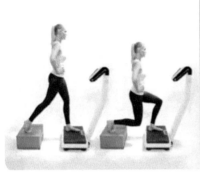

AMPLITUDE **H**
FREQUENCY **H**
60s
REST **30s**

Lunge LEFT

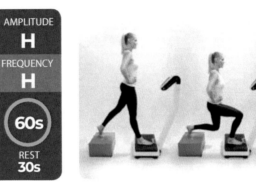

AMPLITUDE **H**
FREQUENCY **H**
60s
REST **30s**

Lunge RIGHT

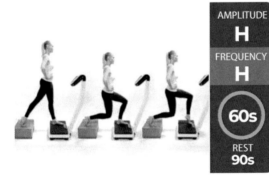

AMPLITUDE **H**
FREQUENCY **H**
60s
REST **90s**

Lunge Calf Raise LEFT

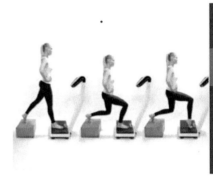

AMPLITUDE **H**
FREQUENCY **H**
60s
REST **90s**

Lunge Calf Raise RIGHT

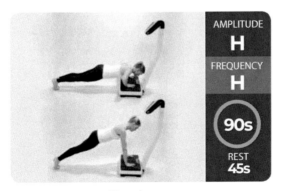

AMPLITUDE **H**
FREQUENCY **H**
90s
REST **45s**

Pushup

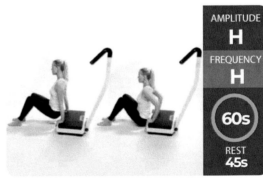

AMPLITUDE **H**
FREQUENCY **H**
60s
REST **45s**

Triceps Dip

Trim, Tight & Toned 3

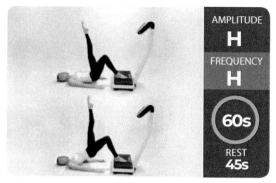

AMPLITUDE **H**
FREQUENCY **H**
60s
REST **45s**

Single leg Bridge LEFT

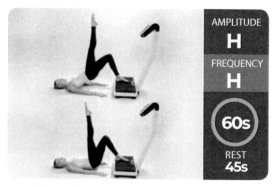

AMPLITUDE **H**
FREQUENCY **H**
60s
REST **45s**

Single leg Bridge RIGHT

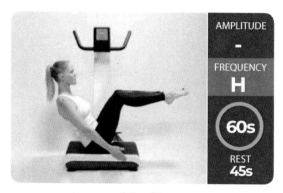

AMPLITUDE **-**
FREQUENCY **H**
60s
REST **45s**

V-sit

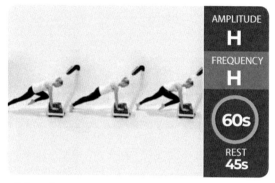

AMPLITUDE **H**
FREQUENCY **H**
60s
REST **45s**

Plank with Mountain Climber

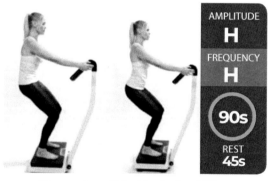

AMPLITUDE **H**
FREQUENCY **H**
90s
REST **45s**

Squat with Pelvic Tilts

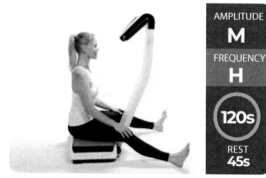

AMPLITUDE **M**
FREQUENCY **H**
120s
REST **45s**

Hamstring Massage

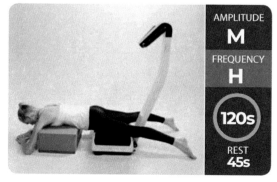

AMPLITUDE **M**
FREQUENCY **H**
120s
REST **45s**

Quadriceps Massage

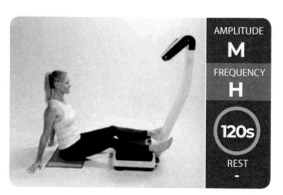

AMPLITUDE **M**
FREQUENCY **H**
120s
REST **-**

Calf Massage

Cellulite Removal

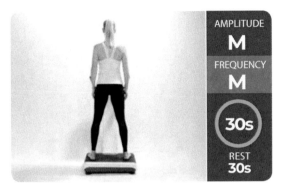
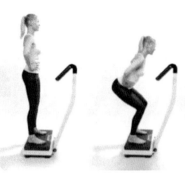
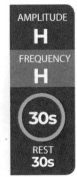

Wide Stance

Mini Squat

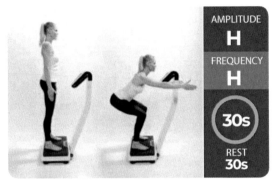
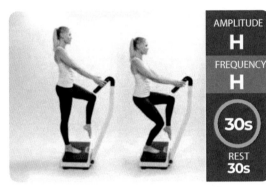

Deep Squat

Single Leg Squat LEFT

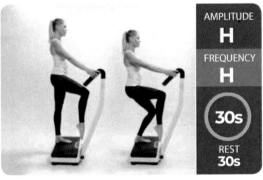
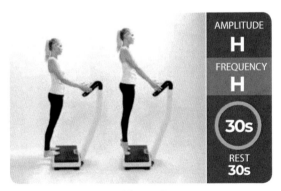

Single Leg Squat RIGHT

Calf Raise

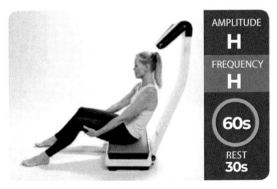
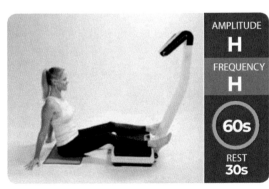

Seated Massage

Calf Massage

Cellulite Removal

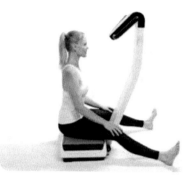

Hamstring Massage

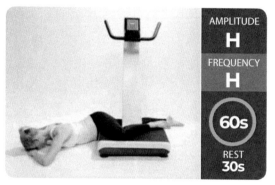

Quadriceps Massage

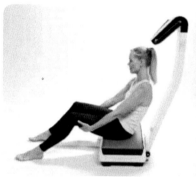
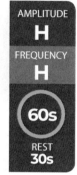

Seated Massage

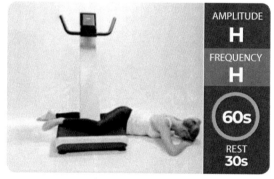
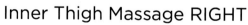

Inner Thigh Massage LEFT

Inner Thigh Massage RIGHT

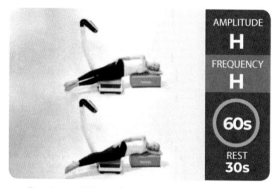

Outer Thigh Massage LEFT

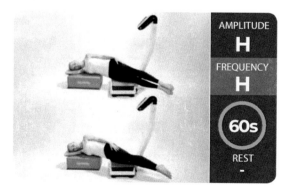

Outer Thigh Massage RIGHT

Pelvic Floor

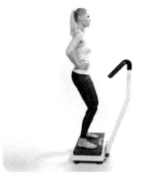

AMPLITUDE
M
FREQUENCY
M
60s
REST
45s

Normal Stance

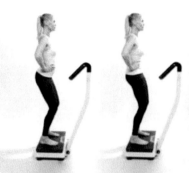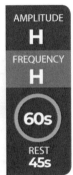

AMPLITUDE
H
FREQUENCY
H
60s
REST
45s

Pelvic Tilts

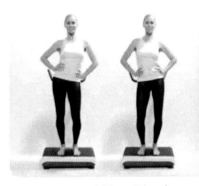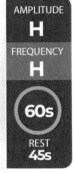

AMPLITUDE
H
FREQUENCY
H
60s
REST
45s

Hip Circles

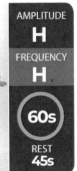

AMPLITUDE
H
FREQUENCY
H
60s
REST
45s

Deep Squat

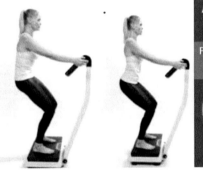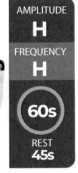

AMPLITUDE
H
FREQUENCY
H
60s
REST
45s

Squat with Pelvic Tilt

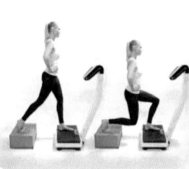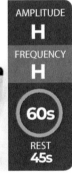

AMPLITUDE
H
FREQUENCY
H
60s
REST
45s

Lunge LEFT

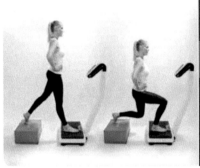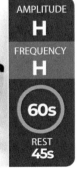

AMPLITUDE
H
FREQUENCY
H
60s
REST
45s

Lunge RIGHT

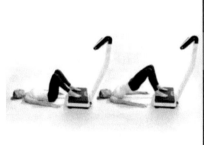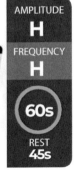

AMPLITUDE
H
FREQUENCY
H
60s
REST
45s

Bridge

Pelvic Floor

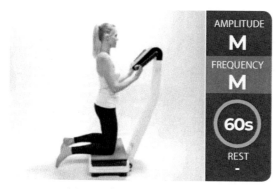

AMPLITUDE
M
FREQUENCY
M
60s
REST
-

Kneeling Kegel's

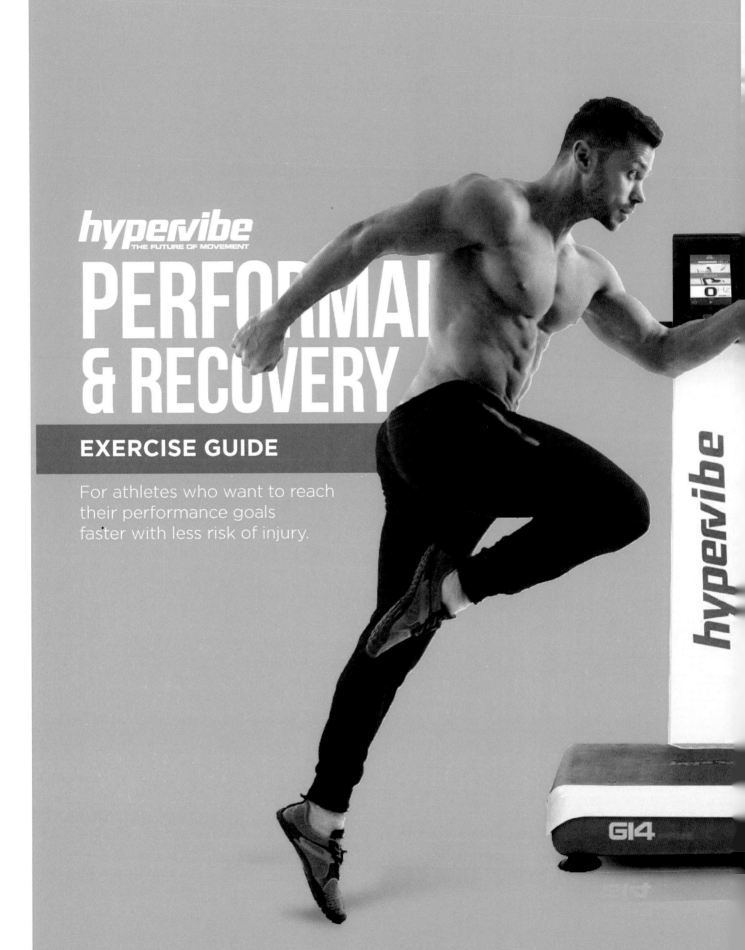

hypervibe
THE FUTURE OF MOVEMENT

PERFORMAN
& RECOVERY

EXERCISE GUIDE

For athletes who want to reach
their performance goals
faster with less risk of injury.

Golf

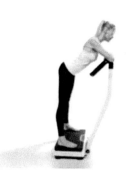

AMPLITUDE **M**
FREQUENCY **M**
120s
REST **30s**

Lumbar Massage

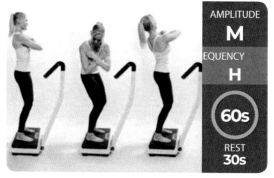

AMPLITUDE **M**
FREQUENCY **M**
60s
REST **30s**

Lumbar Rotation

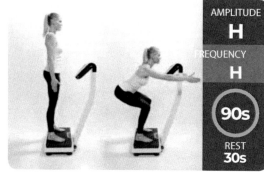

AMPLITUDE **M**
FREQUENCY **H**
60s
REST **30s**

Advanced Rotation

AMPLITUDE **H**
FREQUENCY **H**
90s
REST **30s**

Deep Squat

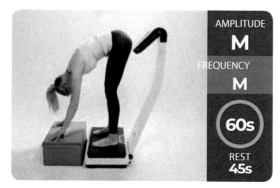

AMPLITUDE **M**
FREQUENCY **M**
60s
REST **45s**

Assisted Hamstring Stretch

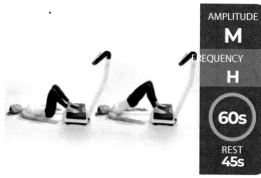

AMPLITUDE **M**
FREQUENCY **H**
60s
REST **45s**

Bridge

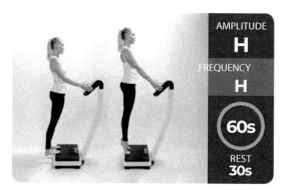

AMPLITUDE **H**
FREQUENCY **H**
60s
REST **30s**

Calf Raise

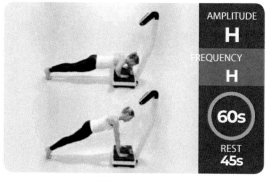

AMPLITUDE **H**
FREQUENCY **H**
60s
REST **45s**

Push Up

Golf

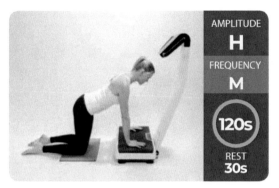

Shoulder Massage

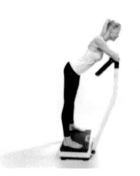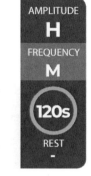

Lumbar Massage

Volleyball & Basketball

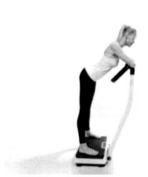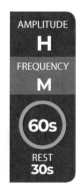

Lumbar Massage

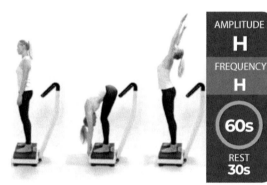

Lumbar Roll

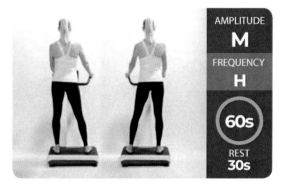

Standing Weight Shift

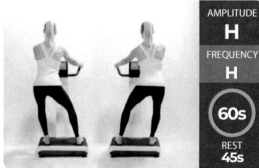

Squat with Weight Shift

Volleyball & Basketball

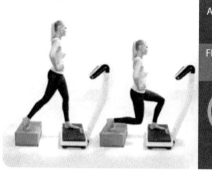

AMPLITUDE H
FREQUENCY H
60s
REST 45s

Lunge LEFT

AMPLITUDE H
FREQUENCY H
60s
REST 45s

Lunge RIGHT

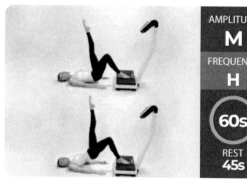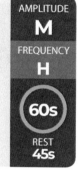

AMPLITUDE M
FREQUENCY H
60s
REST 45s

Single Leg Bridge LEFT

AMPLITUDE M
FREQUENCY H
60s
REST 45s

Single Leg Bridge RIGHT

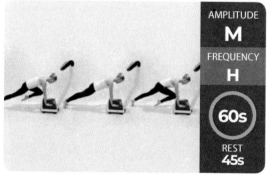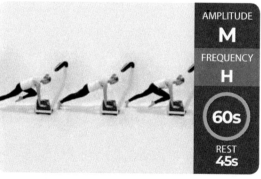

AMPLITUDE M
FREQUENCY H
60s
REST 45s

Plank with Mountain Climber

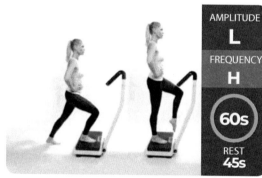

AMPLITUDE L
FREQUENCY H
60s
REST 45s

Step Up with Knee Lift LEFT

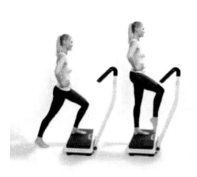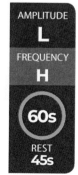

AMPLITUDE L
FREQUENCY H
60s
REST 45s

Step Up with Knee Lift RIGHT

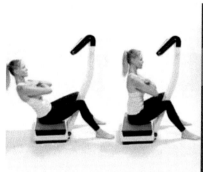

AMPLITUDE -
FREQUENCY H
60s
REST 45s

Abdominal Crunch

Volleyball & Basketball

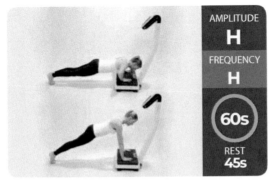

AMPLITUDE	H
FREQUENCY	H
60s	
REST	45s

Push Up

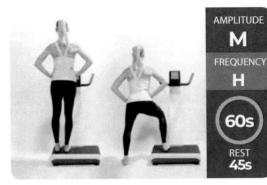

AMPLITUDE	M
FREQUENCY	H
60s	
REST	45s

Lateral Step Up LEFT

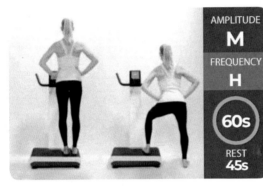

AMPLITUDE	M
FREQUENCY	H
60s	
REST	45s

Lateral Step Up RIGHT

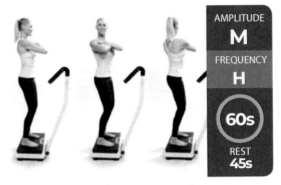

AMPLITUDE	M
FREQUENCY	H
60s	
REST	45s

Lumbar Rotation

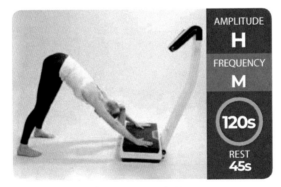

AMPLITUDE	H
FREQUENCY	M
120s	
REST	45s

Downward Dog

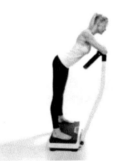

AMPLITUDE	H
FREQUENCY	M
120s	
REST	-

Lumbar Massage

Running

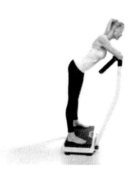

Lumbar Massage

AMPLITUDE **H**
FREQUENCY **M**
60s
REST **30s**

Lumbar Roll

AMPLITUDE **M**
FREQUENCY **H**
60s
REST **30s**

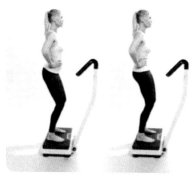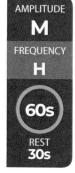

Pelvic Tilts

AMPLITUDE **M**
FREQUENCY **H**
60s
REST **30s**

Squat with Weight Shift

AMPLITUDE **H**
FREQUENCY **H**
60s
REST **45s**

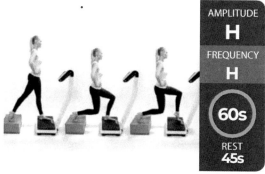

Lunge with Calf Raise LEFT

AMPLITUDE **H**
FREQUENCY **H**
60s
REST **45s**

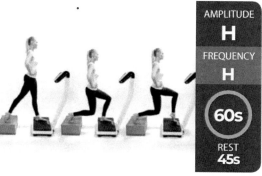

Lunge with Calf Raise RIGHT

AMPLITUDE **H**
FREQUENCY **H**
60s
REST **45s**

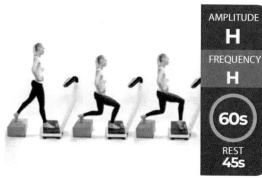

Single Leg Bridge LEFT

AMPLITUDE **M**
FREQUENCY **H**
60s
REST **45s**

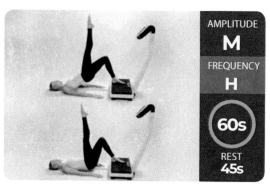

Single Leg Bridge RIGHT

AMPLITUDE **M**
FREQUENCY **H**
60s
REST **45s**

Running

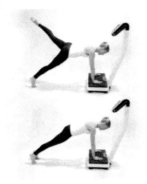
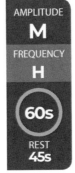

AMPLITUDE **M**
FREQUENCY **H**
60s
REST **45s**

Plank with Hip Extension

AMPLITUDE **L**
FREQUENCY **H**
60s
REST **45s**

Step Up with Knee Lift LEFT

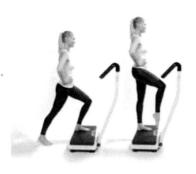
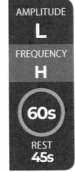

AMPLITUDE **L**
FREQUENCY **H**
60s
REST **45s**

Step Up with Knee Lift RIGHT

AMPLITUDE **-**
FREQUENCY **H**
60s
REST **45s**

Advanced Abdominals

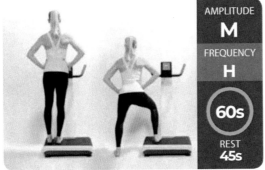
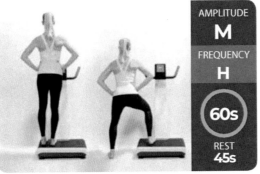
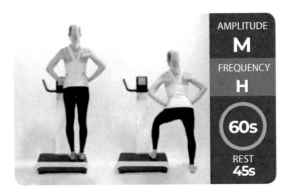

AMPLITUDE **M**
FREQUENCY **H**
60s
REST **45s**

Lateral Step Up LEFT

AMPLITUDE **M**
FREQUENCY **H**
60s
REST **45s**

Lateral Step Up RIGHT

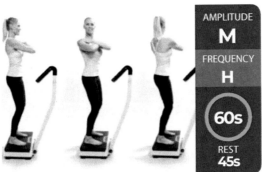
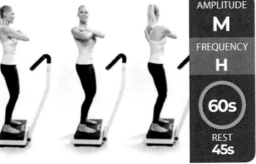
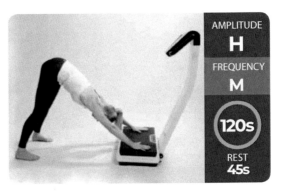

AMPLITUDE **M**
FREQUENCY **H**
60s
REST **45s**

Lumbar Rotation

AMPLITUDE **H**
FREQUENCY **M**
120s
REST **45s**

Downward Dog

Running

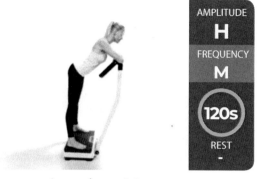

Lumbar Massage

Cycling

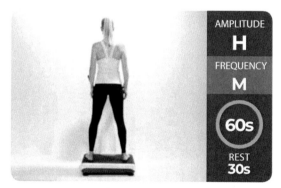

Lumbar Massage

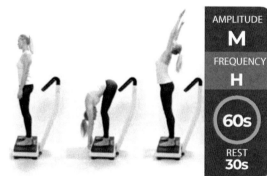

Lumbar Roll

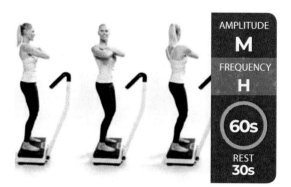

Lumbar Rotation

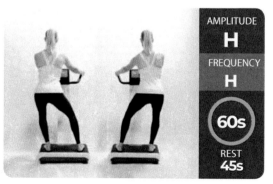

Squat with Weightshift

Cycling

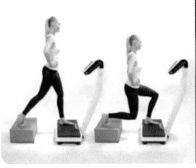

AMPLITUDE H
FREQUENCY H
60s
REST 45s

Lunge LEFT

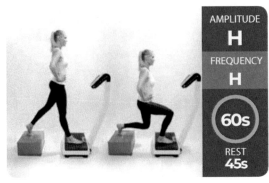

AMPLITUDE H
FREQUENCY H
60s
REST 45s

Lunge RIGHT

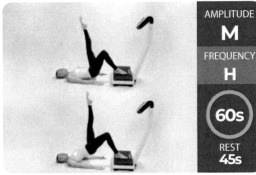

AMPLITUDE M
FREQUENCY H
60s
REST 45s

Single Leg Bridge LEFT

AMPLITUDE M
FREQUENCY H
60s
REST 45s

Single Leg Bridge RIGHT

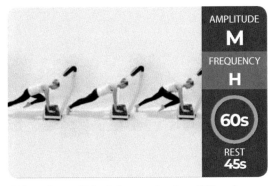

AMPLITUDE M
FREQUENCY H
60s
REST 45s

Plank with Mountain Climber

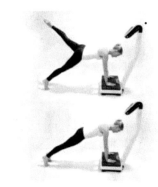
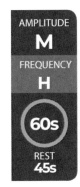

AMPLITUDE M
FREQUENCY H
60s
REST 45s

Plank with Hip Extension

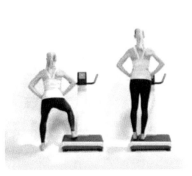
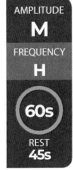

AMPLITUDE M
FREQUENCY H
60s
REST 45s

Step Up LEFT

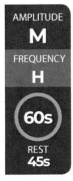

AMPLITUDE M
FREQUENCY H
60s
REST 45s

Step Up RIGHT

Cycling

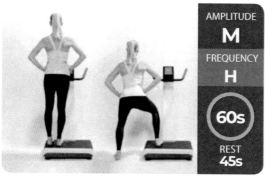

Lateral Step Up LEFT

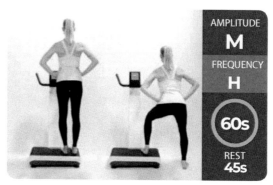

Lateral Step Up RIGHT

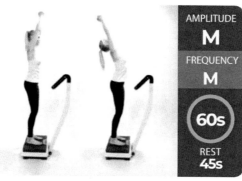

Lumbar Extension

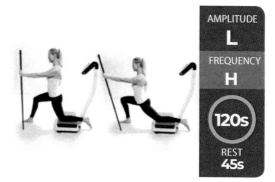

Assisted Hip Flexor Stretch LEFT

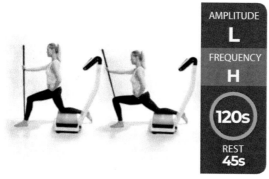

Assisted Hip Flexor Stretch RIGHT

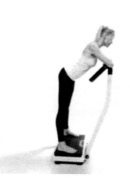

Lumbar Massage

Upper Body Recovery

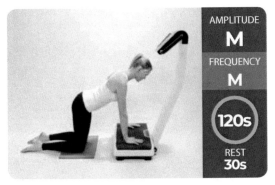

Shoulder Massage

AMPLITUDE **M**
FREQUENCY **M**
120s
REST **30s**

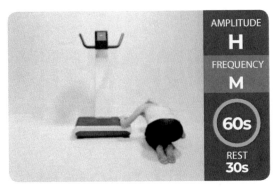

Pectoralis Stretch LEFT

AMPLITUDE **H**
FREQUENCY **M**
60s
REST **30s**

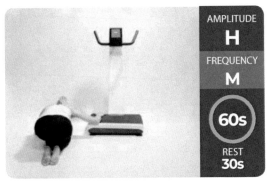

Pectoralis Stretch RIGHT

AMPLITUDE **H**
FREQUENCY **M**
60s
REST **30s**

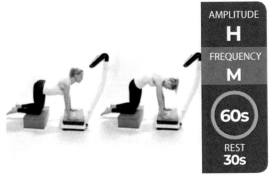

Cat and Camel Stretch

AMPLITUDE **H**
FREQUENCY **M**
60s
REST **30s**

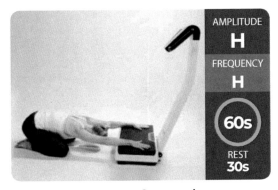

Prayer Stretch

AMPLITUDE **H**
FREQUENCY **H**
60s
REST **30s**

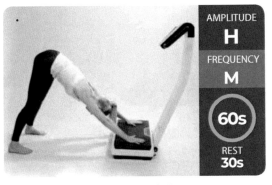

Downward Dog

AMPLITUDE **H**
FREQUENCY **M**
60s
REST **30s**

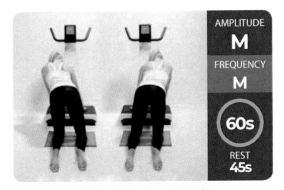

UE Weight Shift

AMPLITUDE **M**
FREQUENCY **M**
60s
REST **45s**

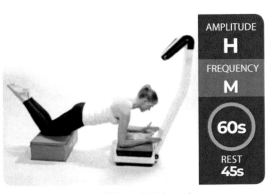

Modified Plank

AMPLITUDE **H**
FREQUENCY **M**
60s
REST **45s**

Upper Body Recovery

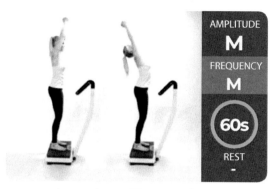

AMPLITUDE **M**
FREQUENCY **M**
60s
REST **-**

Lumbar Extension

Lower Body Recovery

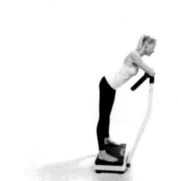

AMPLITUDE **H**
FREQUENCY **M**
120s
REST **30s**

Lumbar Massage

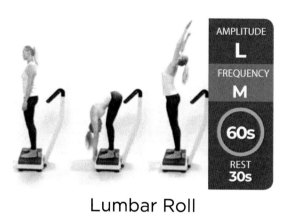

AMPLITUDE **L**
FREQUENCY **M**
60s
REST **30s**

Lumbar Roll

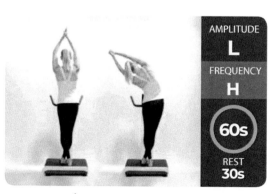

AMPLITUDE **L**
FREQUENCY **H**
60s
REST **30s**

ITB/TFL Stretch LEFT

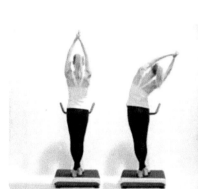
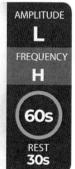

AMPLITUDE **L**
FREQUENCY **H**
60s
REST **30s**

ITB/TFL Stretch RIGHT

Lower Body Recovery

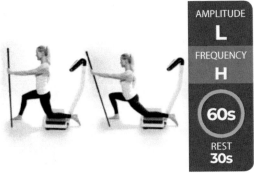

Assisted Hip Flexor Stretch LEFT

AMPLITUDE L
FREQUENCY H
60s
REST 30s

Assisted Hip Flexor Stretch RIGHT

AMPLITUDE L
FREQUENCY H
60s
REST 30s

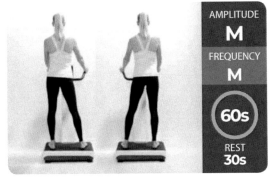

Standing Weight Shift

AMPLITUDE M
FREQUENCY M
60s
REST 30s

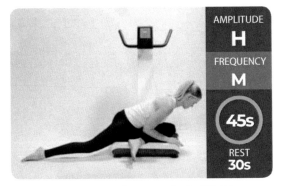

Pigeon Stretch LEFT

AMPLITUDE H
FREQUENCY M
45s
REST 30s

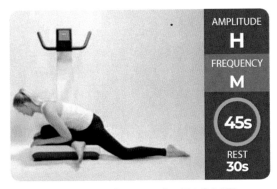

Pigeon Stretch RIGHT

AMPLITUDE H
FREQUENCY M
45s
REST 30s

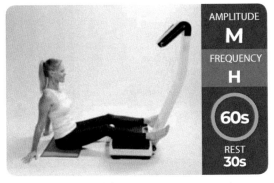

Calf Massage

AMPLITUDE M
FREQUENCY H
60s
REST 30s

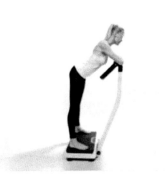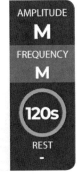

Lumbar Massage

AMPLITUDE M
FREQUENCY M
120s
REST -

hypervibe
THE FUTURE OF MOVEMENT

RELIEVE & REVIVE

EXERCISE GUIDE

For people who want relief from aches &
pains, and to improve their health and
wellbeing.

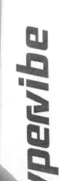

Low Back Relief

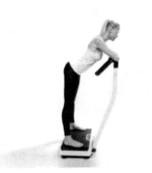

AMPLITUDE H
FREQUENCY M
90s
REST 30s

Lumbar Massage

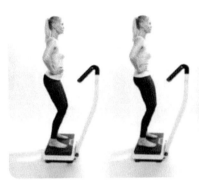
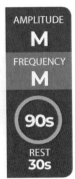

AMPLITUDE M
FREQUENCY M
90s
REST 30s

Pelvic Tilts

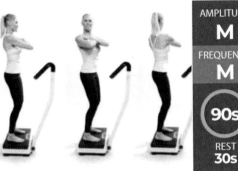
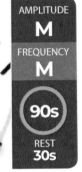

AMPLITUDE M
FREQUENCY M
90s
REST 30s

Lumbar Rotation

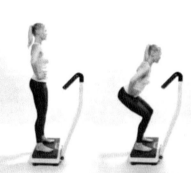
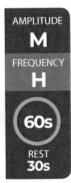

AMPLITUDE L
FREQUENCY M
90s
REST 30s

Assisted Hamstring Stretch

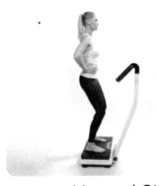
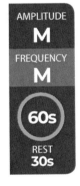

AMPLITUDE M
FREQUENCY M
60s
REST 30s

Normal Stance

AMPLITUDE M
FREQUENCY H
60s
REST 30s

Mini Squat

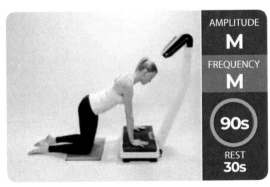

AMPLITUDE M
FREQUENCY M
90s
REST 30s

Shoulder Massage

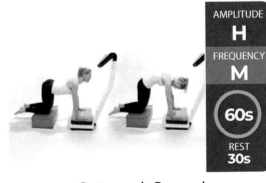

AMPLITUDE H
FREQUENCY M
60s
REST 30s

Cat and Camel

Low Back Pain

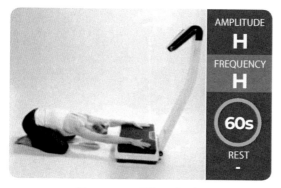

Prayer Stretch

Lymphatic

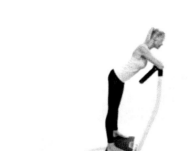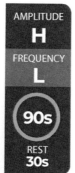

Lumbar Massage

Calf Massage

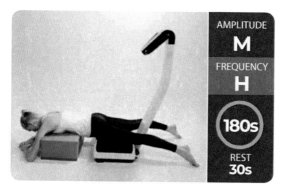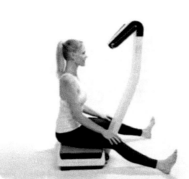

Quadriceps Massage

Hamstring Massage

Lymphatic

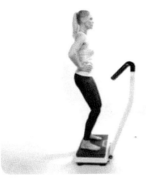 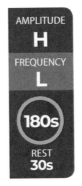

Normal Stance

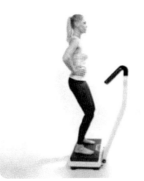 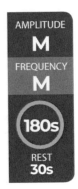

Normal Stance

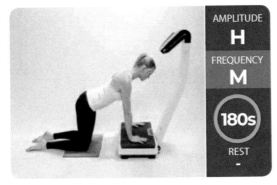

Shoulder Massage

Massage

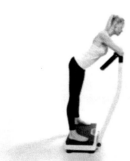 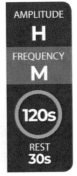

Lumbar Massage

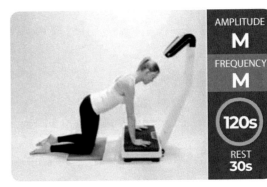

Shoulder Massage

Massage

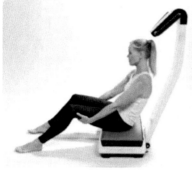

AMPLITUDE	FREQUENCY		REST
-	H	90s	30s

Seated Massage

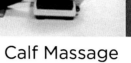

AMPLITUDE	FREQUENCY		REST
M	H	90s	30s

Calf Massage

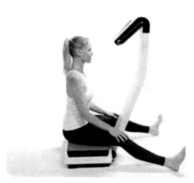

AMPLITUDE	FREQUENCY		REST
M	H	90s	30s

Hamstring Massage

AMPLITUDE	FREQUENCY		REST
M	H	90s	30s

Quadriceps Massage

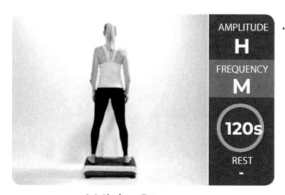

AMPLITUDE	FREQUENCY		REST
H	M	120s	-

Wide Stance

Neck Relief

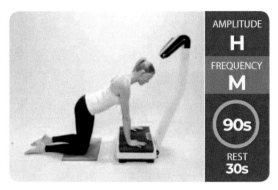

AMPLITUDE	H
FREQUENCY	M
90s	
REST	30s

Shoulder Massage

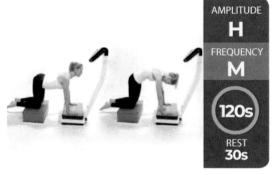

AMPLITUDE	H
FREQUENCY	M
120s	
REST	30s

Cat and Camel Stretch

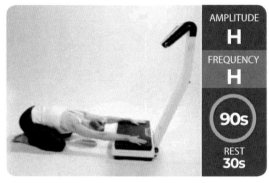

AMPLITUDE	H
FREQUENCY	H
90s	
REST	30s

Prayer Stretch

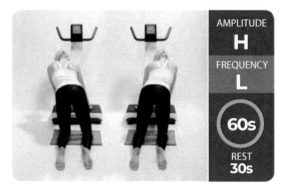

AMPLITUDE	H
FREQUENCY	L
60s	
REST	30s

UE Weightshift

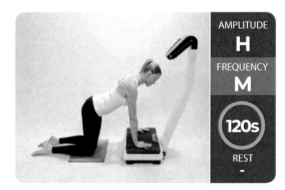

AMPLITUDE	H
FREQUENCY	M
120s	
REST	-

Shoulder Massage

Functional Stability

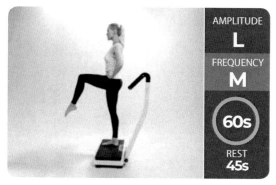

Single Leg Standing LEFT

AMPLITUDE L
FREQUENCY M
60s
REST 45s

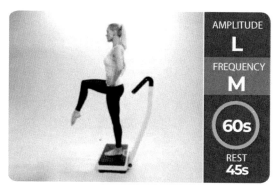

Single Leg Standing RIGHT

AMPLITUDE L
FREQUENCY M
60s
REST 45s

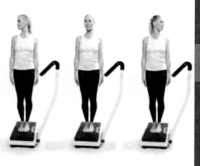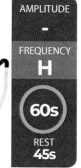

Narrow Side Stance with Head Turn

AMPLITUDE -
FREQUENCY H
60s
REST 45s

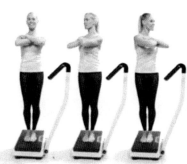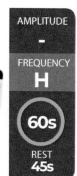

Narrow Side Stance with Rotation

AMPLITUDE -
FREQUENCY H
60s
REST 45s

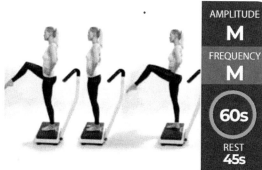

Alternating Knee Lift

AMPLITUDE M
FREQUENCY M
60s
REST 45s

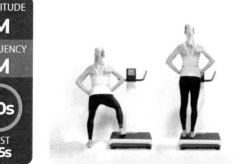

Step Up LEFT

AMPLITUDE H
FREQUENCY M
45s
REST 45s

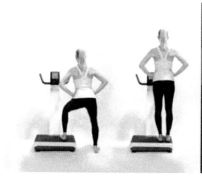

Step Up RIGHT

AMPLITUDE H
FREQUENCY M
45s
REST 45s

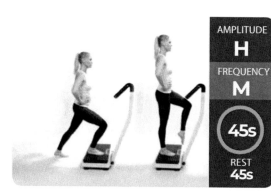

Step Up with Knee Lift LEFT

AMPLITUDE H
FREQUENCY M
45s
REST 45s

Functional Stability

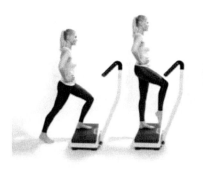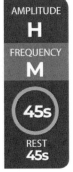

Step Up with Knee Lift RIGHT

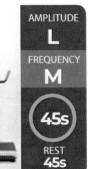

Lateral Step Up LEFT

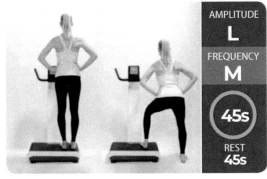

Lateral Step Up RIGHT

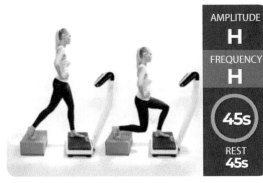

Lunge LEFT

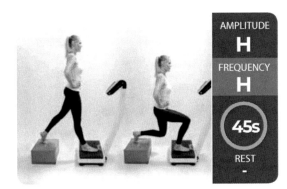

Lunge RIGHT

Functional Stability Progression

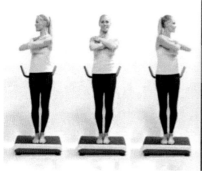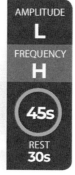

AMPLITUDE **L**
FREQUENCY **H**
45s
REST **30s**

Narrow Stance with Rotation

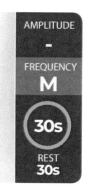

AMPLITUDE **-**
FREQUENCY **M**
30s
REST **30s**

Tandem Side Stance

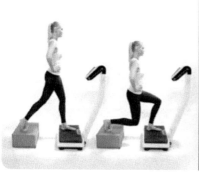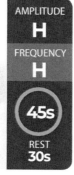

AMPLITUDE **H**
FREQUENCY **H**
45s
REST **30s**

Lunge LEFT

AMPLITUDE **H**
FREQUENCY **H**
45s
REST **30s**

Lunge RIGHT

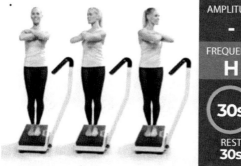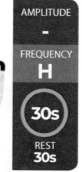

AMPLITUDE **-**
FREQUENCY **H**
30s
REST **30s**

Narrow Side Stance with Rotation

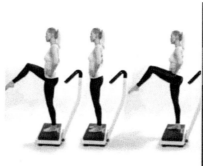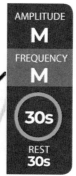

AMPLITUDE **M**
FREQUENCY **M**
30s
REST **30s**

Alternating Knee Lift

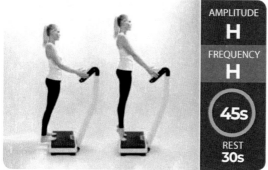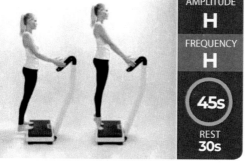

AMPLITUDE **H**
FREQUENCY **H**
45s
REST **30s**

Calf Raise

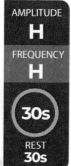

AMPLITUDE **H**
FREQUENCY **H**
30s
REST **30s**

Step Up with Knee Lift LEFT

Functional Stability Progression

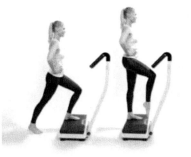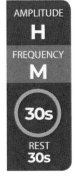

AMPLITUDE **H** FREQUENCY **M** **30s** REST **30s**

Step Up with Knee Lift RIGHT

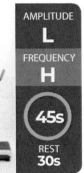

AMPLITUDE **L** FREQUENCY **H** **45s** REST **30s**

Lateral Step Up LEFT

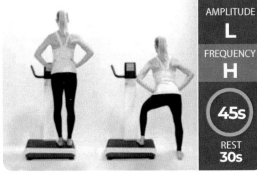

AMPLITUDE **L** FREQUENCY **H** **45s** REST **30s**

Lateral Step Up RIGHT

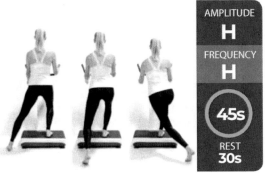

AMPLITUDE **H** FREQUENCY **H** **45s** REST **30s**

3 Way Lunge LEFT

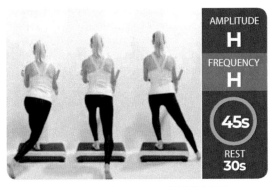

AMPLITUDE **H** FREQUENCY **H** **45s** REST **30s**

3 Way Lunge RIGHT

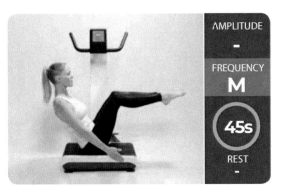

AMPLITUDE **-** FREQUENCY **M** **45s** REST **-**

V-sit

DISCLAIMER

Statements made in this guide have not been evaluated by the Food and Drug Administration. This guide not intended to diagnose, treat, cure, or prevent any disease. Information provided in this guide is not a substitute for individual medical advice. The results via this guide may vary based on individual users and are not guaranteed.

hypervibe
THE FUTURE OF MOVEMENT

Made in the USA
Las Vegas, NV
22 December 2024

15295301R00090